ACCLAIM GARNERED BY PREVIOUS EDITIONS OF THE
NEW YORK TIMES BESTSELLER

THE NEW GLUCOSE REVOLUTION

∎

"Forget *Sugar Busters*. Forget *The Zone*. If you want the real scoop on how carbohydrates and sugar affect your body, read this book by the world's leading researchers on the subject. It's the authoritative, last word on choosing foods to control your blood sugar."

—JEAN CARPER, best-selling author of *Miracle Cures, Stop Aging Now!* and *Food: Your Miracle Medicine,* on *The Glucose Revolution*

"The concept of the glycemic index has been distorted and bastardized by popular writers and diet gurus. Here, at last, is a book that explains what we know about the glycemic index and its importance in designing a diet for optimum health."

—ANDREW WEIL, MD, on *The Glucose Revolution*

"Clear, accessible, and authoritative information about the glycemic index. An exciting, new approach to preventing obesity, diabetes, and heart disease—written by internationally recognized experts in the field."

—DAVID LUDWIG, MD, PhD, Director, Obesity Program, Children's Hospital, Boston, and coauthor, *Ending the Food Fight: Guide Your Child to a Healthy Weight in a Fast Food/Fake Food World*, on *The New Glucose Revolution*

"Mounting evidence indicates that refined carbohydrates and high glycemic index foods are contributing to the escalating epidemics of obesity and type 2 diabetes worldwide. This dietary pattern also appears to increase the risk of heart disease and stroke. The skyrocketing proportion of calories from added sugars and refined carbohydrates in westernized diets portends a future acceleration of these trends. *The Glucose Revolution* challenges traditional doctrines about optimal nutrition and the role of carbohydrates in health and disease. Brand-Miller and colleagues are to be congratulated for an eminently lucid and important book that explains the science behind the glycemic index and provides tools and strategies for modifying diet to incorporate this knowledge. I strongly recommend the book to both health professionals and the general public who could use this state-of-the-art information to improve health and well-being."

—JOANN E. MANSON, MD, DrPH, Professor of Medicine, Harvard Medical School, and Codirector of Women's Health, Division of Preventive Medicine, Brigham and Women's Hospital

"Here is at last a book explaining the importance of taking into consideration the glycemic index of foods for overall health, athletic performance,

and in reducing the risk of heart disease and diabetes. The book clearly explains that there are different kinds of carbohydrates that work in different ways and why a universal recommendation to "increase the carbohydrate content of your diet" is plainly simple and scientifically inaccurate. Everyone should put the glycemic index approach into practice."
—ARTEMIS P. SIMOPOULOS, MD,
senior author of *The Omega Diet* and *The Healing Diet* and President, The Center for Genetics, Nutrition, and Health, Washington, DC,
on *The Glucose Revolution*

"*The Glucose Revolution* is nutrition science for the 21st century. Clearly written, it gives the scientific rationale for why all carbohydrates are not created equal. It is a practical guide for both professionals and patients. The food suggestions and recipes are exciting and tasty."
—RICHARD N. PODELL, MD, MPH, Clinical Professor,
Department of Family Medicine, UMDNJ–Robert Wood Johnson Medical School, and coauthor of *The G-Index Diet: The Missing Link That Makes Permanent Weight Loss Possible*

"The glycemic index is a useful tool which may have a broad spectrum of applications, from the maintenance of fuel supply during exercise to the control of blood glucose levels in diabetics. Low glycemic index foods may prove to have beneficial health effects for all of us in the long term. *The Glucose Revolution* is a user-friendly, easy-to-read overview of all that you need to know about the glycemic index. This book represents a balanced account of the importance of the glycemic index based on sound scientific evidence."
—JAMES HILL, PhD, Director, Center for Human Nutrition,
University of Colorado Health Sciences Center

"*The New Glucose Revolution* summarizes much of the recent development of dietary glycemic index and load in a highly readable format. The authors are able researchers and respected leaders in the nutrition field. Much that is discussed in this book draws directly from their years of experimental and observational research. The focus on dietary intervention and prevention strategies in every day eating is an especially laudable feature of this book. I recommend this book most highly as an indispensable source of good nutrition."
—SIMIN LIU, MD, MS, MPH, ScD,
Professor, Department of Epidemiology, UCLA School of Public Health

"As a coach of elite amateur and professional athletes, I know how critical the glycemic index is to sports performance. *The New Glucose Revolution* provides the serious athlete with the basic tools necessary for getting the training table right."
—JOE FRIEL, coach, author, consultant

The NEW
GLUCOSE
Revolution

THE ALL-NEW 3RD EDITION
Completely Revised and Expanded

THE ALL-NEW 3RD EDITION
Completely Revised and Expanded

The NEW

GLUCOSE

Revolution

The Authoritative Guide to
THE GLYCEMIC INDEX
—the Dietary Solution
for Lifelong Health

Jennie Brand-Miller, PhD
Thomas M. S. Wolever, MD, PhD
Kaye Foster-Powell, M Nutr & Diet
Stephen Colagiuri, MD

MARLOWE & COMPANY
NEW YORK

THE NEW GLUCOSE REVOLUTION: *The Authoritative Guide to the Glycemic Index—the Dietary Solution for Lifelong Health*—3rd Edition

Text copyright © 1996, 1998, 1999, 2002, 2003, 2007 Dr. Jennie Brand-Miller, Kaye Foster-Powell, Dr. Stephen Colagiuri, Dr. Thomas M. S. Wolever

Published by
Marlowe & Company
An Imprint of Avalon Publishing Group, Incorporated
245 West 17th Street • 11th Floor
New York, NY 10011-5300

This is a completely revised edition of *The New Glucose Revolution*,
published in North America by Marlowe & Company in 2003
(and in a previous edition, as *The Glucose Revolution*, in 1999).
This edition is published by arrangement with Hachette Livre Australia.

The GI symbol Ⓖ, a trademark of the University of Sydney that is recognized in Australia, the United States, and in other countries, is a public health initiative that provides consumers with a credible signpost to healthier food choices using the internationally recognized benefits of GI and sound nutrition. More information about the program is at www.gisymbol.com. All other trademarks are the property of their respective owners. Avalon Publishing Group, Inc. is not associated with any product or vendor mentioned in this book.

Library of Congress Cataloging-in-Publication Data
The new glucose revolution : the authoritative guide to the glycemic index : the dietary solution for lifelong health / Jennie Brand-Miller ... [et al.] ; recipes by Kaye Foster-Powell and Lisa Lintner. — 3rd ed., completely rev. and expanded.
p. cm.
Includes bibliographical references and index.
ISBN-13: 978-1-56924-258-2 (trade pbk.)
ISBN-10: 1-56924-258-5 (trade pbk.)
1. Glycemic index. 2. Carbohydrates in human nutrition. I. Brand-Miller, Jennie, 1952–
QP701.N49 2007
613.2'83—dc22
2006032624

9 8 7 6 5 4 3 2 1

Designed by Pauline Neuwirth, Neuwirth & Associates, Inc.

Printed in the United States of America

Contents

The **NEW**

GLUCOSE
Revolution

THE ALL-NEW 3RD EDITION
Completely Revised and Expanded

Introduction

*T*his book is the definitive guide to the glycemic index, the now universally recognized way to distinguish how different carbohydrates affect your blood glucose levels. The glycemic index (which we will often abbreviate as GI) can help you choose the right *amount* of carbohydrate and the right *sort* of carbohydrate for your health and well-being—not only at the meals you eat today, but at every meal, every day. *Eating the right kind of carbohydrates can positively affect your health today—and over the course of your entire life*. That was the fundamental message of the original edition of this book, first published eleven years ago. Now, more than a decade later, that message is more relevant to more people than ever before. You probably know that your blood glucose levels rise and fall throughout the day, helping determine how you feel and how your body functions. ("Blood sugar" and "blood glucose" mean essentially the same thing. Throughout this book we will use the term *blood glucose*, which is scientifically more precise.) Grounded in more than twenty-five years of research, *The New Glucose Revolution* thoroughly explains the relationship between carbohydrates and your blood glucose and how the connection between the two affects your health, both immediately and later in life.

■ Who Can Use ■
The New Glucose Revolution?

Now more than ever, the glycemic index is for **everybody**, **every day**, at **every meal**. The glycemic index—as well as its newer companion concept, the glycemic load, about which you may have heard, and which we will also discuss—is relevant for everyone. People concerned about their heart health—who are risk for heart disease or heart attack or who are at risk for or already have the metabolic syndrome (insulin resistance syndrome, formerly known as syndrome X)—will greatly benefit by putting into practice the findings and recommendations of *The New Glucose Revolution*.

So, too, will women with polycystic ovarian syndrome (PCOS), and everyone interested in controlling their weight.

The New Glucose Revolution is essential reading for everyone with diabetes and prediabetes, offering an alternative to hard-to-follow, misguided, and often counterproductive dietary restrictions. Many people with type 1 or type 2 diabetes find that despite doing all the right things, their blood glucose levels fluctuate excessively and/or remain too high. If you or someone you are caring for has diabetes, *The New Glucose Revolution* will give you the knowledge and know-how to choose the right kind of carbohydrate for optimum blood glucose control.

It's also for those who want to prevent these conditions in the first place, and to improve their overall health. Particularly in the last decade, research conducted by scientists throughout the world has underscored—not only to us, but to many individual experts and health-related authorities worldwide—that the glycemic index of foods has implications for everybody. It is truly a glucose revolution, in that a growing mountain of research on the GI has permanently changed the way we understand carbohydrates and their effect on our bodies.

The *New Glucose Revolution* Helps People:

- with type 1 diabetes
- with type 2 diabetes
- with prediabetes (who may have been told they have "a touch of diabetes" or have impaired glucose tolerance)
- with gestational diabetes (diabetes during pregnancy)
- with hypoglycemia, or low blood glucose
- who are overweight or obese
- who are at a normal weight but have too much fat around the middle (abdominal overweight)
- with higher than desirable blood glucose levels
- with high levels of triglycerides and low levels of HDL cholesterol
- with metabolic syndrom (insulin resistance syndrome, formerly known as syndrome X)
- with polycystic ovarian syndrome (PCOS)
- with nonalcoholic fatty liver (NAFL) disease or nonalcoholic steatohepatitis (NASH)
- who want to prevent all of the above and live a healthier life.
- New research also indicates that a low GI diet may also be helpful in delaying or preventing age-related macular degeneration (AMD).

The reason *The New Glucose Revolution* can help you is simple: high blood glucose levels are a key—and undesirable—characteristic of all of these conditions, with both short- and long-term adverse effects. *The New Glucose Revolution* will show you how to better manage your blood glucose levels by understanding and making the best use of the glycemic index.

■ An Overview of *The New Glucose Revolution*— ■ and What's New in This Edition

This third edition of *The New Glucose Revolution* presents the most comprehensive, up-to-date information about the GI, including exciting new research and commentary from real people whose lives have been changed by adopting a low glycemic index, or "low-GI," diet approach. (Over many years we've received thousands of letters and e-mails with useful feedback from readers all over the world regarding earlier editions of this book and our other books.)

As we'll detail throughout this book, the scientific evidence to support the central role the GI can play in your health has now been firmly established. In fact, it goes much further than we ever imagined when we all variously began our research (which dates as far back as the early 1980s, when the glycemic index was first developed, as we'll describe shortly). We share our own and other researchers' scientific findings with you—and what these findings mean for your life and well-being.

Among the features that are new to this third edition of *The New Glucose Revolution* are:

▶ All of the very latest findings (as of time of publication) regarding the glycemic index and diabetes, heart disease, weight loss, and nonalcoholic fatty liver disease

▶ An introduction to and overview of glycemic load

▶ Insight into weight gain in pregnancy, gestational diabetes, diseases such as polycystic ovarian syndrome (PCOS, closely linked to insulin resistance), and celiac disease

▶ Real-life stories of people who have dramatically improved their health by making the switch to low-GI eating, every day, at every meal

▶ A clear rationale for choosing our low-GI diet plan from among the many different diet plans that circulate today

▶ An all-new chapter on eating the low-GI way for vegetarians

▶ Dozens of new recipes

▶ An extensive glossary, with nearly 100 key terms, now clearly defined, all in one place

▶ The newest published GI values for a wide variety of recently tested foods, including such favorites as wild blueberries, maple syrup, and pomegranate juice

■ Making the Most of *The New Glucose* ■ *Revolution*—A Quick Guide to Its Organization

Part 1 presents a complete overview of the glycemic index—what it is, how it works—and about carbohydrates, more broadly—specifically, why we need them and how much carbohydrate you should be eating. We explain the importance of being conscious of the types of carbohydrates and fats you eat—no matter what the proportions of protein, fat, and carbohydrate. We also discuss the glycemic load, a newer GI-related nutrition tool.

In part 2 we break down exactly how the glycemic index—and specifically, a low-GI diet—can aid in weight control, as well as how it can help manage and prevent a variety of health conditions and concerns, including type 1 diabetes, type 2 diabetes, polycystic ovarian syndrome (PCOS), heart disease, the metabolic syndrome (insulin resistance syndrome, formerly known as syndrome X), gestational diabetes, hypoglycemia, and sports performance. We also discuss how the glycemic index applies to healthy eating for children.

Part 3 answers more than forty of the most commonly asked questions about the glycemic index. If you've wondered about something relating to the GI, you should find the answer here.

Part 4 is your guide to low-GI eating. We outline our seven key dietary guidelines, explain how you can easily make the switch to eating the right kinds of carbs; what to keep stocked in your pantry, refrigerator, and freezer; and quick-and-easy ideas for breakfast, lunch, dinner, and between-meal snacks. Part 4 also includes more than forty-five easy and delicious recipes, along with their GI ratings and nutritional analysis. We also discuss how vegetarians can adhere to a low-GI diet.

You'll find the actual GI values for more than five hundred foods in the updated and much improved tables in part 5, the most comprehensive and authoritative list of GI values for different foods. You'll find foods listed alphabetically as well as according to types (breads, fruits, vegetables, etc.); the information includes not only the GI value and amount of carbohydrate per serving, but also their glycemic load. We've added the foods that we're often asked about—meat, fish, cheese, broccoli, avocados, and others—even though many of them don't contain carbohydrate and their GI equals zero.

Finally, we end with a brand-new A-to-Z glossary (throughout the book, we boldface words that are defined there), as well as our references section.

A key note about the references section: we are scientists, medical doctors, and clinicians (to read more about us, see "Meet the Medical Doctors, Scientists, and Clinicians Behind *The New Glucose Revolution*," on page 347). We value the research and clinical data that forms the backbone of this book and is behind every one of our recommendations. Every recommendation we make in this book has scientific validity. The references underscore our grounding in scientific research, and they're there for all of you who like to familiarize yourselves with original scientific findings and may want to trace our ideas back to their original sources.

We make this promise to you: with *The New Glucose Revolution* you'll discover and come to understand that a way of eating for lifelong health that is easy, delicious, wonderfully varied, does not depend on deprivation, and is truly satisfying on many levels. Welcome to this important revolution—now more than twenty-five years in the making—and one we're delighted to share with you.

A Crash Course in Current Scientific Thinking— Ten Big Myths About Food and Health Dispelled

THROUGHOUT THIS BOOK we'll dispel a number of myths about food and carbohydrates. To start you off, we bust the ten most common myths about food (sugar and other carbs, especially) and health.

MYTH 1 ■ Starchy foods such as bread and pasta are fattening.
FACT ■ Most starchy foods are bulky and nutritious. They fill you up and stave off hunger pangs—which means they can actually help with, rather than hinder, weight loss. The key, as with all foods, is to be choosy about what kinds of starchy foods you're eating, watch your portion size, and make sure you're not consuming more calories than you burn each day.

MYTH 2 ■ Sugar causes diabetes.
FACT ■ Today, an absolute consensus exists among health researchers

and scientists specializing in diabetes that sugar in food does not cause diabetes. Type 1 diabetes (formerly known as insulin-dependent or juvenile diabetes) is an autoimmune condition triggered by unknown environmental factors. Type 2 diabetes (formerly known as non-insulin-dependent diabetes) is largely inherited, but lifestyle factors such as a lack of exercise or being overweight increase the risk of developing it. Foods that produce high blood glucose levels may increase the risk of type 2 diabetes, but sugar, as you'll learn, has a more moderate effect than many starches, especially refined and highly processed ones.

MYTH 3 ■ Sugar is the worst thing for people with diabetes.

FACT ■ People with diabetes used to be advised to avoid sugar at all costs. But research shows that moderate consumption of refined sugar (2–3 tablespoons—around 40 grams, or 1½ oz) a day doesn't compromise blood glucose control. This means people with diabetes can choose foods that contain refined sugar or even use small amounts of table sugar. Overprocessed flours and grains and saturated fat are of greater concern for people with diabetes.

MYTH 4 ■ All starches are slowly digested in the intestine.

FACT ■ Not so. Most starch, especially that in refined-grain products, is digested in a flash, causing a faster and more severe increase in blood glucose than many sugar-containing foods.

MYTH 5 ■ Hunger pangs are inevitable if you want to lose weight.

FACT ■ High-carbohydrate foods, especially those with a low GI (rolled oats and pasta, for example), can keep you feeling full, often until you're ready to eat your next meal.

MYTH 6 ■ Foods high in fat are more filling.

FACT ■ Studies show that high-fat foods are among the least filling. That's why, in part, it's so easy to passively overconsume high-fat foods like potato chips.

MYTH 7 ■ Sugar is fattening.

FACT ■ Sugar has no special fattening properties. It is no more likely to be turned into fat than any other type of carbohydrate. Yes, sugar is often present in foods high in energy (or calories) and fat (cakes and cookies, for instance). But it's the total calories in those energy-dense foods (a concept we'll explain more fully; see page 72), not the sugar, that contribute to the body's creation of fat and excess weight.

MYTH 8 ■ Starches are best for optimum athletic performance.
FACT ■ In many instances, starchy foods (like potatoes or rice) are too bulky to eat in the quantities needed for active athletes. Sugars (from a range of sources, including dairy food and fruit) can help increase carbohydrate intake.

MYTH 9 ■ Diets high in sugar are less nutritious.
FACT ■ Studies have shown that diets high in sugar (from a range of sources, including dairy foods and fruit) often have higher levels of micronutrients, including calcium, riboflavin, and vitamin C, than low-sugar diets.

MYTH 10 ■ Sugar goes hand in hand with dietary fat.
FACT ■ Yes, many foods high in fat are also high in sugar—think chocolate, full-fat ice cream, cakes, cookies, and pastries. But most high-sugar diets are actually low in fat, and vice versa. The reason: most sources of fat in our diet are not sweetened (e.g., potato chips, French fries, steak), while most sources of sugar contain no fat (e.g., soft drinks and sweetened juice drinks).

PART 1

What Is the Glycemic Index

The Glycemic Index—A Brief Overview ■ Exactly How Does the Glycemic Index Work? ■ What's Wrong with Today's Diet? ■ Carbohydrates—The Big Picture: What They Are, Why We Need Them, How We Digest Them ■ How Much Carbohydrate Do You Need?

▪1▪

The Glycemic Index—
A Brief Overview

*T*oday **we know** that not all **carbohydrate** foods are created equal. In fact, they can behave quite differently in our bodies. The **glycemic index**, or **GI**, is a measure of carbohydrate quality. It is (a) a ranking that describes how much the carbohydrates (sugars and starches) in individual foods affect **blood glucose levels**; and (b) a physiologically based measure—a comparison of carbohydrates based on their immediate impact on your blood glucose levels. (By physiologically based, we mean that it is determined by testing in real people.)

Foods containing carbohydrates that break down quickly during digestion have the highest GI values. Their blood glucose response is fast and high—in other words, the **glucose** in the bloodstream increases rapidly. Foods that contain carbohydrates that break down slowly, releasing glucose gradually into the bloodstream, have low GI values. They can keep you feeling full longer, help you achieve and maintain a healthy weight, and provide you with more consistent energy throughout the day. They can also have a major effect on the way your body functions and whether or not you develop health problems.

For most people, under most circumstances, foods with low GI values have advantages over those with high GI values. But there are exceptions: some athletes can benefit from ingesting high-GI foods during and after competition (which we explain in chapter 12), and high-GI foods are also useful in the treatment of hypoglycemia (covered in chapter 8).

> HIGH-GI FOODS cause spikes in your glucose levels, whereas low-GI foods encourage gentle increases and decreases.

■ The Early Development ■ of the Glycemic Index

The glycemic index was developed in 1980–1981 by Dr. David J. A. Jenkins, now a professor in the department of nutritional sciences at the University of Toronto, where he is also Canada Research Chair in Nutrition and Metabolism. Jenkins wanted to determine which foods were best for people with diabetes. At the time, the diet most often recommended for people with diabetes was based on a system of carbohydrate exchanges. Each exchange, or portion of food, contained the same amount of carbohydrate. The exchange system assumed that all starchy foods produced the same effect on blood glucose levels—even though some earlier studies had already proven this was not correct. Jenkins was one of the first researchers to challenge the use of exchanges, and to investigate how individual foods actually affected blood glucose levels in people.

Jenkins and his colleagues, who included *New Glucose Revolution* coauthor Dr. Thomas M. S. Wolever, tested a large number of foods that people commonly ate. Their results generated some big surprises. First, they found that the starch in foods like bread, potatoes, and many types of rice is in fact digested and absorbed very quickly, not slowly, as had previously been assumed.

Second, scientists found that the sugar in foods such as fruit, chocolate, and ice cream did not produce more rapid or prolonged rises in blood glucose, as had always been thought. The truth was that most of the sugars in foods produced quite moderate blood glucose responses, lower than that of most starches.

Because Jenkins's approach was so logical and systematic, yet also contrary to prevailing current thinking and recommendations, it attracted an enormous amount of attention from other scientists and medical researchers upon the publication of his original scientific paper in the *American Journal of Clinical Nutrition* in March 1981.

Since that time, medical researchers and scientists around the world, including the authors of this book, have tested the effect of many foods on blood glucose levels, thus further developing Jenkins's concept of classifying carbohydrates based on what he had termed the glycemic index (GI). Today, thanks to years of testing, we know the GI values of hundreds of different foods. The detailed tables in part 5 give the GI values of a range of foods, including many tested by *New Glucose Revolution* coauthors Dr. Jennie Brand-Miller at the University of Sydney and Dr. Thomas M. S. Wolever (who is still a colleague of Dr. Jenkins's), at the University of Toronto.

■ A Growing Body of Research Supports ■ the Glycemic Index

The GI was a very controversial topic among researchers and health authorities for many years, for a variety of reasons. Initially, some criticism was justified. For example, in the early days there was no evidence that the GI values of single foods could influence the resulting blood glucose levels of the entire meals in which they were consumed—or even that low-GI foods could bring long-term benefits. There were no studies of the glycemic index's reproducibility, or of the consistency of GI values from one country to another. Many of the early studies used only healthy volunteers rather than those with relevant health conditions. What's more, there was no evidence that the results could be applied to people with diabetes.

But today, countless studies from major leading medical institutions and research universities around the world have repeatedly demonstrated that the glycemic index holds up in tests (in scientific terms, it is reproducible) and is a clinically proven tool in its application to appetite, diabetes, and coronary health. To date, studies in the United Kingdom, France, Italy, Sweden, Australia, and Canada have proved the value of the glycemic index. Moreover, diabetes organizations in

Canada, Australia, and the United Kingdom have endorsed using the glycemic index in the dietary management of diabetes.

Overall, health authorities in the United States have been slower to embrace the GI than many of their counterparts elsewhere in the developed world. This may be the result of a number of factors, including the fact that the earliest research into the glycemic index was conducted outside the United States. In the diabetes realm, the American Diabetes Association (ADA) has for many years endorsed dietary recommendations premised on the idea of **carbohydrate counting** (which assumes that all starchy foods produced the same effect on blood glucose levels), an idea that the GI dramatically dispels.

However, in their 2006 nutrition recommendations for the management of diabetes, the ADA noted, "The use of the glycemic index/glycemic load may provide a modest additional benefit over that observed when total carbohydrate is considered alone."

And things may be changing even more broadly in the United States. The *American Dietary Guidelines*, a revised version of which was jointly published in January 2005 by the U.S. Departments of Agriculture (USDA) and of Health and Human Services, made no mention of the GI, but they do emphasize the nutritional virtues of eating whole grains and fruits and vegetables. In addition, the Harvard School of Public Health and the Children's Hospital in Boston recommend the glycemic index, even for healthy people.

More than one research study has shown that a low-GI diet is easy to follow—meaning you're more likely to stick with it than you would other regimes. In fact, one study from Children's Hospital in Boston reported that study participants found a low-GI diet regimen easier to maintain than diets that restrict fat or carbohydrates.

■ Just What Was So Revolutionary about the ■ Development of the GI?

Before the development of the GI, the nature of **carbohydrates** was described by their chemical structure: *simple* or *complex*. Sugars were simple, and starches were complex, only because sugars were small molecules and starches were big ones. It was assumed that complex carbohydrates, such as **starches**, because of their large size, would be slowly digested and absorbed and would therefore cause only a small and gradual rise in blood glucose levels. Simple **sugars**, on the other hand, were assumed to be digested and absorbed quickly, producing a rapid increase in blood glucose.

A GI Success Story

"FOR YEARS, I tried everything I could to lose weight so I'd look better and stop feeling tired all the time. But nothing worked, and I was always hungry! Finally, a friend recommended I pick up *The New Glucose Revolution*. I read it and slowly started applying the principles of a low-GI diet (e.g., I ate bran cereal instead of white bread in the morning, pasta instead of a sandwich, fruit for a snack instead of a muffin) to my diet. Slowly, but surely—and with a bit of exercise—the weight came off, and I ultimately lost 22 pounds! I'm no longer hungry all the time, and I have so much more energy. Best of all, I can't believe how easy it is to consistently follow a low-GI diet. This is not a fad but a way of eating that I will always stick to."

—Sarah

Prior to David Jenkins's research in the early 1980s, scientists had conducted simple experiments on solutions of raw starches and pure sugars and had drawn conclusions about real foods from them. It is important to note, however, that these conclusions did not apply to real foods eaten at real meals. For fifty years the conclusions from these experiments were taught to every medical and biochemistry student as "fact." These "facts," and the assumptions on which they were based, are what the GI so definitively overturned.

Thanks to the GI, we now know that the whole concept of "simple" versus "complex" carbohydrates does not tell us anything about how the carbohydrates in food affect blood glucose levels in the body. The rise in blood glucose after meals cannot be predicted simply on the basis of a simple versus complex chemical structure. In other words, the old distinctions that were long made between starchy foods (complex carbohydrates) and sugary foods (simple carbohydrates) have no useful application when it comes to blood glucose levels—and all of the health issues that relate to them.

The glycemic index describes the type of carbohydrate in foods. It indicates their ability to raise your blood glucose levels. Foods with a high GI value contain carbohydrates that cause a dramatic rise in blood glucose levels, while foods with a low GI value contain carbohydrates that have much less of an impact.

• 2 •

Exactly How Does the Glycemic Index Work?

■ How Scientists Measure the Glycemic Index ■

A food's GI value must be determined physiologically in human subjects (we call this *in vivo testing*) according to an internationally standardized method. Currently, fewer than ten facilities around the world test GI values by following the now standard international testing protocol. (You may hear about *in vitro* [test tube] methods, but these are shortcuts, that may be useful for manufacturers developing new products, but may not reflect the true GI of a food.) These facilities include:

North America:
▶ Glycemic Index Laboratories, Inc., Toronto, Canada (www.gilabs.com)

Australia and New Zealand:
▶ The University of Sydney's Glycemic Index Research Service (SUGIRS), Sydney, Australia (www.glycemicindex.com)

- International Diabetes Institute, Melbourne, Australia (www.idi.org.au)
- Glycaemic Index Otago, University of Otago, New Zealand (www.glycemicindex.otago.ac.nz)

UK and Europe:
- Leatherhead Food International, Surrey, UK (www.lfra.co.uk)
- Oxford Brookes University, Oxford, UK (www.brookes.ac.uk/bms/research/nfsg/index.html)
- Hammersmith Food Research Unit, Hammersmith Hospital, London, UK (www.foodresearch.co.uk)
- Reading Scientific Services Limited (RSSL), Reading, UK (www.rssl.com)
- Biofortis, Nantes, France (www.biofortis.fr)
- NutriScience BV, Maastricht, Netherlands (www.nutri-science.nl)
- Oy Foodfiles Ltd., Kuopio, Finland (www.foodfiles.com)

■ The GI Testing Protocol ■

In the standard method of GI testing, ten volunteers consume a 50-gram carbohydrate portion of the test food (e.g., 1 cup of rice) on one occasion and a 50-gram carbohydrate portion of the reference food on another occasion. Pure glucose dissolved in water is the usual reference food and its GI is set at 100. The test is carried out in the morning after an overnight fast. The food is eaten within ten to twelve minutes, and blood glucose levels are measured at frequent intervals over the next two hours.

Each volunteer's blood glucose response to the test food is then plotted on a graph and compared with his or her response to the reference food (figure 1); that graphic response is referred to as the **area under the curve**—the exact percentages are calculated using a computer program.

If the test food response area (i.e., the area under the curve) is only 40 percent of the reference food, then the GI of the test food is 40. Not everyone will give exactly the same number, of course, but the law of averages applies. If we tested them over and over again, they will all tend to congregate around the same number. Because each person is his or her own control, testing foods in volunteers with diabetes gives approximately the same GI values as testing normal subjects.

In practice, the average result in the group of ten healthy individuals is the published GI value of the food.

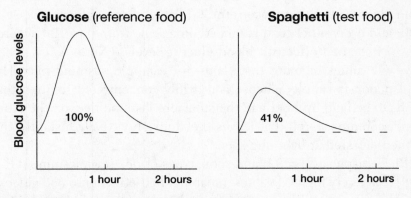

FIGURE 1. Measuring the glycemic index value of a food.

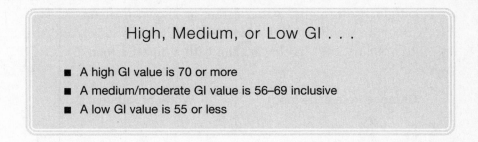

A food's GI value cannot be predicted from its composition, carbohydrate content, or even the GI values of related foods. The only way to know a food's GI value is to test it, following the standardized methodology we've just described.

Unfortunately, there is no easy, inexpensive substitute test. Now, more than two decades after the GI's inception, we and others around the world have determined definitive GI values for more than five hundred foods; these values appear in part 5 of this book, as well as in annually updated editions of *The New Glucose Revolution Shopper's Guide to GI Values* and at our Web site, www.glycemicindex.com.

The higher a food's GI value (or simply, its GI), the higher the blood glucose levels are after an individual consumes that food. Foods with a high GI usually reach a higher peak ("glycemic spike"), but sometimes blood glucose levels remain moderately high over the entire two-hour period; white bread is a good example of this (see figure 2).

Why is glucose used as the reference food? Pure glucose itself produces one of the greatest effects on blood glucose levels. GI testing has shown that *most* foods have less effect on blood glucose levels than glucose. For that reason, the GI value of pure glucose is set at 100, and every other food is ranked on a scale from 0 to 100 according to its actual effect on blood glucose levels. (Note: A few foods have GI values of more than 100—for example, jasmine rice. The explanation is simple: glucose is a highly concentrated solution that tends to be held up briefly in the stomach. Jasmine rice, on the other hand, contains starch that leaves the stomach virtually instantly and is then digested at lightning speed.)

Rice Krispies (GI = 82) and some types of rice (e.g., jasmine [GI = 109]) have very high GI values, meaning their effect on blood glucose levels is almost as high as that of an equal amount of pure glucose. Foods with a low GI value (such as lentils, GI = 26–48) show a flatter blood glucose response when eaten, as shown in figure 3. That means that the resulting peak blood glucose level is lower, and the return to baseline levels is slower than with a high-GI food.

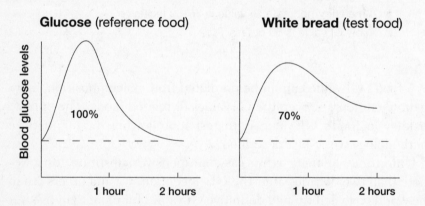

FIGURE 2. The effect of pure glucose (50 grams) and white bread (50-gram carbohydrate portion) on blood glucose levels.

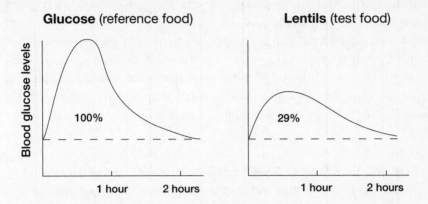

Glucose (reference food)   **Lentils** (test food)

FIGURE 3. The effect of pure glucose (50 grams) and lentils (50-gram carbohydrate portion) on blood glucose levels.

■ Why Low-GI Foods Are a Smart Choice ■

For most people, low-GI foods have advantages over high-GI foods. The slow digestion and gradual increase and decrease in blood glucose responses after eating a low-GI food helps control blood glucose levels in people with diabetes or glucose intolerance. This effect benefits healthy people as well, because it reduces the secretion of the hormone **insulin** over the course of the whole day. (We discuss this in greater detail in chapters 3 and 9.) Plus, slower digestion helps to delay hunger pangs—meaning you're less likely to overeat or make poor food choices as the result of hunger, which can promote weight loss if you're overweight.

Lower glucose levels over the course of the day also improve heart health. High insulin levels resulting from a regular diet of high-GI carbs promote high blood fats, high blood glucose, and high blood pressure, thus increasing the risk of heart attack. Keeping your blood glucose levels on an even keel helps ensure that your blood vessels remain elastic and supple, reducing the formation of fatty streaks and plaques that cause **atherosclerosis**—known more widely as hardening of the arteries. And good blood glucose control means your body is less likely to form blood clots in the arteries, which can precipitate a heart attack. The fluctuation of blood glucose levels also increases inflammation: fluctuating glucose levels stresses cells and triggers inflammatory responses.

You don't have to eat only low-GI foods to benefit. Studies show that when a low- and a high-GI food are combined in one meal (e.g., lentils and rice), the overall blood glucose response is intermediate. You can keep both your glucose and insulin levels lower over the course of the whole day if you choose at least one low-GI food at each meal.

FOR MOST PEOPLE, low-GI foods have advantages over high-GI foods. The slow digestion and gradual increase and decrease in blood glucose responses after eating a low-GI food helps control blood glucose levels in people with diabetes or glucose intolerance. Plus, slower digestion helps to delay hunger pangs—meaning you're less likely to overeat or make poor food choices as the result of hunger, which can promote weight loss if you're overweight.

■ Can the GI Be Applied to the Meals ■ You Eat Each Day?

Criticism of the GI has focused on unpredictable outcomes of blood glucose values in meals because of variations in fat, protein, and fiber levels. Most of our meals consist of a variety of foods—not just a single food. Even though GI values are originally derived from testing single foods in isolation, we and other scientists have found that it is possible to predict the blood glucose response for a meal that consists of several foods with different GI values.

Concerned about the methodology of recent studies showing unpredictable responses, we and our coresearchers at the University of Toronto's Department of Nutritional Sciences and the University of Sydney's Human Nutrition Unit conducted studies with mixed meals on two groups of healthy subjects in Toronto and Sydney. We had previously done much smaller studies. We revisited the question, using more meals and variety in two different centers with judiciously selected foods. This time, fourteen different test meals were used in Sydney and Toronto, and the food combinations reflected typical breakfast choices, such as juice and bagels with cream cheese.

Despite the variations in food, blood glucose responses remained consistent with GI measures. In fact, we were startled by the degree of predictability. The carbohydrate, fat, and protein composition of the meals varied over a wide spectrum. The glucose responses varied over a fivefold range, and 90 percent of the variation was explained by the amount of carbohydrate in the meal and the GI values of the foods as given in published GI tables. We found that the GI works just as predictably whether subjects consume a single portion of one item or a normal meal; we reported these findings in the June 2006 issue of the *American Journal of Clinical Nutrition*.

■ How Do We Calculate the Overall ■ GI Value of a Meal, Menu, or Recipe?

The GI value of a meal is not the sum of the GI values of each food in the meal, nor is it simply an average of their GI values. The GI of a meal, menu, or recipe consisting of a variety of carbohydrate foods is a weighted average of the GI values of each food. The weighting is based on the proportion of the total carbohydrate contributed by each food.

Over the years, many readers—researchers and clinicians in the nutrition field, as well as laypeople—have asked us to explain how to calculate the total GI of a meal. So for their benefit, and for the more curious among you, we take a moment to walk you through two brief examples.

To calculate the GI of a mixed meal, you need to know the GI of the carbohydrate foods in the meal (information we provide in the tables in part 5), plus the total carbohydrate content of the meal and the contribution of each food to the total carbohydrate. You will find this information in food-composition tables or nutrient-analysis computer programs. The following calculations may look complicated—and in fact, in practice you don't need to make these sorts of calculations to adopt the low-GI way of eating, but dietitians and nutrition researchers sometimes have to.

Example 1. Let's look at a snack of peaches (GI = 42) and ice cream (GI = 37–49). Depending on the amounts of each food, we could calculate the total content of these carbohydrates from food-composition tables. Let's say the meal contains 60 grams of carbohydrate, with 20 grams provided by the peaches and 40 grams by the ice cream. For the purposes of this calculation, we're using low-fat vanilla ice cream (GI = 46).

To estimate the GI value of this dish, we multiply the GI value of peaches by their proportion of the total carbohydrate:

$$42 \times 20 \div 60 = 14$$

and multiply the GI value of ice cream by its proportion of the total carbohydrate:

$$46 \times 40 \div 60 = 31$$

We then add these two figures to give a GI value for this dish of 45.

Example 2. Another scenario, for the classic combination of beans and rice: if half the carbohydrate in the mixed meal comes from a food with a GI value of 30 (e.g., black beans) and the other half from a rice with a GI value of 80, then the mixed meal will have a GI of 55, determined as follows: (50% of 30) + (50% of 80) = 55.

Our rice-and-beans example demonstrates that it's not necessary to avoid all high-GI foods in order to eat a low-GI diet. Nor is it necessary to calculate the GI value for every meal you eat. Rather, simply choose a low-GI food in place of a higher-GI food. Simply including one low-GI food per meal is enough.

We'll share many more helpful dietary suggestions with you throughout the rest of the book—and part 4 is your guide to low-GI eating.

■ Glycemic Index or Glycemic Load? ■

As we have shown, your blood glucose rises and falls when you eat a meal containing carbohydrate. How high and how long it rises depends on two things: how much carbohydrate you eat and the GI of the carbohydrate you eat. The more carbohydrate you eat, the higher your blood glucose goes. The higher the GI of the food you eat, the higher your blood glucose goes. A small amount of a high-GI food may raise your blood glucose as much as a large amount of a low-GI food. The **glycemic load** (GL), initially developed by researchers at Harvard University, puts together the amount of carbohydrate you eat *and* its GI to help predict how much a serving of food will raise blood glucose. If a serving of food has a GL of 10, that means it will raise blood glucose by as much as 10 grams of glucose.

The GL of a food is a mathematical calculation—determined by multiplying the GI of a particular food by the available carbohydrate content (meaning the carbohydrate content minus fiber) in a particular serving size (expressed in grams), divided by 100. The formula is:

$$GL = (GI \times \text{the amount of carbohydrate}) \text{ divided by } 100.$$

Let's take a single apple as an example. It has a GI of 38 and it contains 15 grams of carbohydrate.

$$GL = 38 \times 15 \div 100 = 6$$

What about a small serving of French fries? Its GI is 75 and it contains 29 grams of carbohydrate.

$$GL = 75 \times 29 \div 100 = 22$$

So we can predict that our fries (GL = 22) will have nearly four times the metabolic effect of an apple (GL = 6). You can think of GL as the amount of carbohydrate in a food "adjusted" for its glycemic impact.

Proponents of the GL—both within the scientific nutrition community and beyond it—think that this concept should be used instead of the GI when comparing foods because it more fully reflects a food's glycemic impact on one's body.

But a word of caution: we don't want people actively avoiding carbs and striving for a diet with the lowest GL possible. That's why we advocate sticking with the GI.

For one thing, GL doesn't distinguish between foods that are low carb (and thus higher in fat and/or protein) or slow carb (that is, low-GI carbs). Some people whose diets have an overall lower GL are consuming *more* fat or protein and fewer carbohydrates of any kind, including healthy, low-GI carbs. Following a low-GL path could mean that you're unnecessarily restricting foods, missing out on nutrients and the other proven benefits of a higher-carbohydrate diet, and thus eating a less healthful diet—one that's too low in carbohydrates and full of the wrong types of fats and proteins.

Research also shows that by choosing carbohydrates by their GI value—and opting primarily for those that are low-GI—you'll get a healthy, safe diet with an appropriate quantity and quality of carbohydrate. In fact, you'll be increasing your intake of nutritional powerhouse foods, including fruits and vegetables, whole grains, and legumes (including beans, chickpeas, and lentils). And by choosing low-GI foods, you'll automatically be eating lower-GL foods, too—so a low-GI diet is a win-win situation.

Yes, a handful of high-GI foods, such as watermelon, have a low GL, but we recommend that you don't keep yourself from eating any fruits or vegetables, other than some potatoes and rices (see "This for That" on page 81).

A word here about portion sizes: some carb-rich foods such as pasta have a low GI but *could* have a high GL if the serving size is large. Portion sizes do count.

■

Think *slow* carbs, not *low* carbs.

■

The Bottom Line about Glycemic Index vs. Glycemic Load

▶ Use the GI to identify your best carbohydrate choices.
▶ Keep your portion size in check to limit the overall GL of your diet.

■ What Determines How High or Low ■ a Food's GI Is?

For many years now scientists have been studying what gives one food a high GI and another one a low GI. That research has generated a huge amount of information, which can be confusing. The following table summarizes the factors that influence the GI value of a food.

The physical state of the starch in a food is by far the most important factor influencing its GI value. This is why advances in food processing over the past two hundred years have had such a profound effect on the overall GI values of the carbohydrates we eat.

Factors That Influence the GI Value of a Food

Factor	Mechanism	Examples of food where the effect is seen
Starch gelatinization	The less gelatinized (swollen) the starch, the slower the rate of digestion.	Al dente spaghetti, oatmeal, and cookies have less gelatinized starch.
Physical entrapment	The fibrous coat around beans and seeds and plant cell walls acts as a physical barrier, slowing down access of enzymes to the starch inside.	Pumpernickel and grainy bread, legumes and barley
High amylose to amylopectin ratio*	The more amylose a food contains, the less water the starch will absorb and the slower its rate of digestion.	Basmati rice and legumes contain more amylose than most cereals.
Particle size	The smaller the particle size, the easier it is for water and enzymes to penetrate.	Finely milled flours have high GI values. Stone-ground flours have larger particles and lower GIs.
Viscosity of fiber	Viscous, soluble fibers increase the viscosity of the intestinal contents, and this slows down the interaction between the starch and the enzymes. Finely milled whole-wheat and rye flours have fast rates of digestion and absorption because the fiber is not viscous.	Rolled oats, beans, lentils, apples, Metamucil.
Sugar	The digestion of sugar produces only half as many glucose molecules as the same amount of starch (the other half is fructose). The presence of sugar also restricts gelatinization of the starch by binding water and reducing the amount of "available" water.	Social Tea biscuits, oatmeal cookies, and some breakfast cereals (Kellogg's Frosted Flakes or Smacks) that are high in sugar have relatively low GI values.
Acidity	Acids in foods slow down stomach emptying, thereby slowing the rate at which the starch can be digested.	Vinegar, lemon juice, lime juice, some salad dressings, pickled vegetables, sourdough bread
Fat	Fat slows down the rate of stomach emptying, thereby slowing the digestion of the starch.	Potato chips have a lower GI value than boiled white potatoes.

* Amylose and amylopectin are two different types of starch.
Both are found in foods, but the ratio varies (see page 22).

■ The Effect of Starch Gelatinization ■
on the Glycemic Index

The **starch** in raw food is stored in hard, compact granules that make it difficult to digest. This is why potatoes would probably give you a stomachache if you ate them raw and why most starchy foods need to be cooked. During cooking, water and heat expand the starch granules to different degrees; some granules actually burst and free the individual starch molecules. (That's what happens when you make gravy by heating flour and water until the starch granules burst and the gravy thickens.)

If most of the starch granules have swollen and burst during cooking, the starch is said to be fully gelatinized. Figure 4, below, shows the difference between raw and cooked starch in potatoes.

The swollen granules and free starch molecules are very easy to digest, because the starch-digesting enzymes in the small intestine have a greater surface area to attack. The quick action of the enzymes results in a rapid, blood glucose increase after consumption of the food (remember that starch is nothing more than a string of **glucose** molecules). As a result, food containing starch that is fully gelatinized will have a very high GI value.

In foods such as cookies, the presence of sugar and fat and very little water makes **starch gelatinization** more difficult, and only about half of the granules will be fully gelatinized. For this reason, cookies tend to have medium GI values.

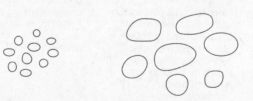

FIGURE 4. The difference between raw (compact granules, left) and cooked (swollen granules, right) starch in potatoes.

■ The Effect of Particle Size ■
on the Glycemic Index

The particle size of a food is another factor that influences starch gelatinization and GI value. Grinding or milling grains reduces particle sizes and makes it easier for water to be absorbed and digestive enzymes to attack the food. This is why many foods made from fine flours tend to have a high GI value. The larger the particle size, the lower the GI value, as figure 5 illustrates.

One of the most significant alterations to our food supply came with the introduction, in the mid-nineteenth century, of steel-roller mills. Not only did they make it easier to remove the fiber from cereal grains, but also the particle size of the starch became smaller than ever before. Prior to the nineteenth century, stone grinding produced quite coarse flours that resulted in slower rates of digestion and absorption.

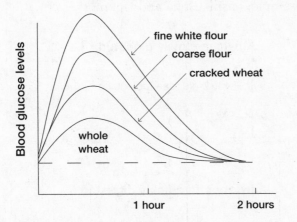

FIGURE 5. The larger the particle size, the lower the GI value.

When starch is consumed in "nature's packaging"—whole intact grains that have been softened by soaking and cooking—the food will have a low GI. For example, cooked barley's GI value is 25; most cooked legumes have a GI of between 30 and 40; and cooked whole wheat berries' GI is 41.

■ The Effect of Amylose and Amylopectin ■ on the Glycemic Index

There are two types of starch in food—*amylose* and *amylopectin*. Researchers have discovered that the ratio of one to the other has a powerful effect on a food's GI value.

Amylose is a straight-chain molecule, like a string of beads. These tend to line up in rows and form tight compact clumps that are harder to gelatinize and therefore harder to digest (see figure 6, below).

Amylopectin, on the other hand, is a string of glucose molecules with lots of branching points, like you'd see in some types of seaweed or a piece of ginger root. Amylopectin molecules are therefore larger and more open, and the starch is easier to gelatinize and to digest. Foods that have little amylose and plenty of amylopectin in their starch have higher GI values—for example, jasmine rice and wheat flour. Foods with a higher ratio of amylose to amylopectin have lower GI values—for example, basmati rice and legumes.

Amylose slowly digested

individual glucose molecules

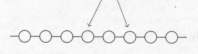

Amylopectin quickly digested

branch point

individual glucose molecules

FIGURE 6. Amylose is a straight-chain molecule that is harder to digest than amylopectin, which has many branching points.

The only whole (intact) grain food with a high GI is low-amylose rice, such as Calrose rice (GI = 83). Low-amylose varieties of rice have starch that is very easily gelatinized during cooking and therefore easily broken down by digestive enzymes. This may help explain why we sometimes feel hungry not long after rice-based meals. However, some varieties of rice (basmati and long-grain white rice) have lower GI values, because they have a higher amylose content than normal rice. Their GI values are in the range of 50 to 59.

Why Does Pasta Have a Low GI Value?

SOMEWHAT SURPRISINGLY, PASTA in any shape or form has a relatively low GI value (30–60). Great news for pasta lovers, but portion size is important. Keep it moderate. In the early days of GI research, we thought that pasta had a low GI value, because the main ingredient was semolina (durum or hard wheat flour), and not finely ground wheat flour. Subsequent research has shown, however, that even pasta made entirely or mostly of plain wheat flour has a low GI value. The reason for the slow digestion rate and subsequent low GI value is the physical entrapment of ungelatinized starch granules in a spongelike network of protein (gluten) molecules in the pasta dough. Pasta and noodles are unique in this regard. Overcooked pasta is very soft and swollen in size and will have a higher GI value than pasta cooked al dente. Adding egg to the dough lowers the GI further by increasing the protein content. Asian noodles such as hokkein, udon, and rice vermicelli also have low to medium GI values.

■ The Effect of Sugar ■
on the Glycemic Index

Table sugar or refined sugar (*sucrose*) has a GI of between 60 and 65. The reason: table sugar is a *disaccharide* (double sugar), composed of one glucose molecule coupled to one fructose molecule. (See chapter 4 for a fuller explanation of the structure of sugars.) **Fructose** is absorbed and taken directly to the liver, where it is immediately oxidized (burned as the source of energy). The blood glucose response to pure fructose is very modest (GI = 19). Consequently, when we consume sucrose, only half of what we've eaten is actually glucose; the other half is fructose. This explains why the blood glucose response to 50 grams of sucrose is approximately half that of 50 grams of corn syrup or *maltodextrins*—where the molecules are all glucose.

Many foods containing large amounts of refined sugar have a GI close to 60. This is the average of glucose (GI = 100) and fructose (GI = 19). It's lower than that of ordinary white bread, with a GI value averaging around 70. Kellogg's Cocoa Puffs, which contains 39 percent sugar, has a GI value of 77, lower than that of Rice Krispies (GI = 82), which contains little sugar.

■

Most foods containing simple sugars do not raise blood glucose levels any more than most complex starchy foods like bread. That fact is one of the key findings of the GI.

■

The sugars that naturally occur in food include lactose, sucrose, glucose, and fructose in variable proportions, depending on the food. On theoretical grounds, it is difficult to predict the overall blood glucose response to a food, because stomach emptying is slowed by increasing the concentration of the sugars.

Some fruits, for example, have a low GI value (grapefruit's GI = 25), while others are relatively high (watermelon = 76). It appears that the higher the acidity of the fruit, the lower the GI value. Consequently, it is not possible to lump all fruits together and say they will have a low GI value, because they are high in fiber. They are not all equal. (For a comparison of all fruits, take a look at the fruit section of the table in part 5, on pages 302 and 303.)

Many foods containing sugars are a mixture of refined and naturally occurring sugars—sweetened yogurt, for example. Their overall effect on blood glucose response is too difficult to predict. This is why we've tested individual foods to determine their GI values rather than guessing or making generalizations about entire food groups.

■ The Effect of Fiber ■
on the Glycemic Index

The effect of **fiber** on the GI value of a food depends on the type of fiber and its viscosity or thickness. Dietary fiber comes from plant foods—it is found in the outer bran layers of grains (corn, oats, wheat, and rice, and in foods containing these grains), fruits and vegetables, and nuts and legumes (dried beans, peas, and lentils). There are two types—soluble and insoluble—and there is a difference.

Soluble fibers are the gel, gum, and often jelly-like components of apples, oats, and legumes. (Psyllium, found in some breakfast cereals and dietary fiber supplements such as Metamucil, is soluble fiber.) These viscous fibers thicken the mixture of food entering the digestive tract. By slowing down the time it takes for the fiber to pass through the stomach and small intestine, foods with high levels of soluble or viscous fiber lower the **glycemic response** to, or glycemic impact on food, which is why legumes, oats, and psyllium have a low GI.

Insoluble fibers are dry and branlike and commonly thought of as roughage. All cereal grains and products made from them that retain the outer layer of the grain are sources of insoluble fiber (e.g., whole-grain bread and All-Bran), but not all foods containing insoluble fiber are low GI. Insoluble fibers will only lower the GI of a food when they exist in their original, intact form—for example, in whole grains of wheat. Here they act as a physical barrier, delaying access of digestive enzymes and water to the starch within the cereal grain. Finely ground wheat fiber, such as in whole-wheat bread, has no effect whatsoever on the rate of starch digestion and subsequent blood glucose response. Breakfast cereals made with whole-wheat flours will also tend to have high GI values unless there are other ingredients in the food that will lower the GI.

The Glycemic Index Was Never Meant to Be Used in Isolation

AT FIRST GLANCE it might appear that some high-fat foods, such as chocolate, seem a good choice simply because they have a low GI value. But this is absolutely not the case. A food's GI value was never meant to offer the only criterion by which it is judged as fit to eat. Large amounts of fat (and protein) in food tend to slow the rate of stomach emptying and therefore the rate at which foods are digested in the small intestine. High-fat foods will therefore tend to have lower GI values than their low-fat equivalents. For example, potato chips have a lower GI value (54) than potatoes baked without fat (77). Many cookies have a lower GI value (55–65) than bread (70). But clearly, in these instances, a lower GI value doesn't translate into a better, healthier choice. Saturated fat in these foods will have adverse effects on coronary health that are far more significant than the benefit of lower blood glucose levels. These foods should be treated as "indulgences," for special occasions, rather than as part of a regular diet.

We are not recommending that you avoid all fats. But just as there are differences in the nature of carbohydrates in foods (what we refer to as the quality, conveyed as the GI value), there are differences in the quality of fats. You should be as choosy about the fats you eat as you are about carbohydrates. Healthy fats, such as the omega-3 polyunsaturated fats, are not only good for you, but they also help to lower the blood glucose response to meals. On the other hand, trans-fatty acids and saturated fats increase your risk of obesity, heart disease, and other serious health conditions.

■ The Effect of Acid ■ on the Glycemic Index

Several research findings over the last decade have indicated that a realistic amount of vinegar or lemon juice in the form of a salad dressing consumed with a mixed meal has significant blood glucose–lowering effects.

As little as 4 teaspoons of vinegar in a vinaigrette dressing (4 teaspoons vinegar + 2 teaspoons oil) taken with an average meal lowered blood glucose by as much as 30 percent. Our research shows that lemon juice is just as powerful. Vinegar or lemon juice may also be used in marinades or sauces.

These findings have important implications for people with diabetes or who are at risk for diabetes, coronary heart disease, or the metabolic syndrome (see chapters 7–9).

The effect appears to be related to the acidity, because some other organic acids (like lactic acid and propionic acid) also have a blood glucose–lowering effect, but the degree of reduction varies with the type of acid.

Blood Glucose and the GI at a Glance

BLOOD GLUCOSE IS the amount of glucose, or sugar, in your blood. It changes throughout the day depending on several factors, most notably what you eat, and it can have a profound effect on your health— your mood, how hungry you are, and whether you develop conditions such as diabetes.

- Your body's blood glucose response to a meal is primarily determined by the meal's carbohydrate content. Both the quantity and quality of carbohydrates in food influence the rise in blood glucose that you experience.
- Carbohydrates that break down quickly during digestion have high GI values. Their blood glucose response is fast and high.
- Carbohydrates that break down slowly, releasing glucose gradually into the bloodstream, have low GI values. In comparison to foods with high GI values, these are more desirable for optimal health.

■

A LOW-GI MEAL TIP: Having a salad prepared with vinegar or lemon juice with your meal, especially a high-GI meal, will help keep your blood glucose under control.

■

Sourdough breads, in which lactic acid and propionic acid are produced by the natural fermentation of starch and sugars by the yeast starter culture, also can reduce levels of blood glucose and insulin by 22 percent compared to normal bread. In addition, studies show that there's higher **satiety**—that is, people feel fuller and more satisfied—associated with breads that have decreased rates of digestion and absorption, like sourdough. There's significant potential to lower your blood glucose and insulin and increase satiety with sourdough breads, so incorporating them into your diet is a smart choice. (We discuss the concept of satiety more fully in chapter 6.)

▪ 3 ▪

What's Wrong
with Today's Diet?

*Y*ou may be wondering, *What's wrong with the way I eat now?* It's
possible that you already follow a balanced, nutrient-dense diet
that emphasizes whole foods and low-GI carbs. But the simple truth
is that the majority of North Americans do not; our culture makes it
all too easy to avoid or stray from a healthful regime. That's why it's so
important to have a concrete, working knowledge of how to eat for
optimum well-being.

We didn't always eat the way we do today. During the Paleolithic
period, humans were hunter-gatherers, consuming the animals and
plants found in their natural environment. Our ancestors were fussy
about which parts of animals they ate. They preferred the hind legs of
the largest animals and the females over the males because they contained more fat and were therefore juicier and more flavorful. They
also enjoyed organ meats—liver, kidneys, brains—foods that are
extremely rich sources of nutrients.

As humans evolved, they became more and more carnivorous.
From the latest studies of modern hunter-gatherer diets, it appears

that they obtained about two-thirds of their energy intake from animal foods (including fish and seafood) and only one-third from plant foods. Although they ate more protein and less carbohydrate than we do now, their fat intake, interestingly, was roughly the same as now—but the type of fat was primarily healthy unsaturated fat rather than unhealthy saturated fat (which we'll discuss shortly). This is because the fat of wild animals, including their organs, has much higher proportions of unsaturated fat than what's typically found in the farmed animals we consume today. Our predecessors' carbohydrate intakes were lower, because the main plant foods they had available were fruits and vegetables rather than cereals. Wheat, rice, and other cereal grains were largely absent until after the emergence of agriculture and the domestication of crops and animals (sometimes called the Neolithic revolution), which began some ten thousand years ago.

So why does this matter to you? Because these findings have strong implications for current dietary recommendations. Although our ancestors ate large amounts of meat when it was available, they also ate large amounts of plant foods (leaves, berries, nuts), which would have been gathered every day, ensuring that their overall diet was both naturally low GI and low GL. It doesn't mean that we all need to eat large amounts of meat to be healthy, but it does imply that the types and amount of **protein**, **carbohydrate**, and **fat** in our diet need to be carefully considered.

Beginning about ten thousand years ago, when we became farmers growing crops rather than hunter-gatherers, our diet changed dramatically (albeit gradually). Starch entered the human diet, in a big way, for the first time; large quantities of harvested cereal grains tipped the human diet ratio from being more animal to more plant. Those plants were whole-grain cereals like wheat, rye, barley, oats, corn, and rice. Legumes (beans), starchy roots and tubers, and fruits and berries also contributed to the now higher-carbohydrate intake of our ancestors. Food preparation was simple: grinding food between stones and cooking it over the heat of an open fire. The result was that although we were eating a high-carbohydrate diet, all the carbohydrates in our food were digested and absorbed slowly; thus, the effects of these foods on our blood glucose were gradual and relatively small.

This diet was ideal because it provided slow-release energy that helped to delay hunger pangs and provided fuel for working muscles long after a meal had been eaten. It was also easy on the insulin-pro-ducing cells in the pancreas.

Over the centuries, flours were ground more and more finely, and bran was separated completely from white flour. With the advent of high-speed roller mills in the nineteenth century, it was possible to pro-duce white flour so fine that it resembled talcum powder in appearance and texture. These fine white flours were—and are—highly prized because they make soft bread and delicious, airy cakes and pastries.

As incomes grew, the foods commonly eaten by our ancestors—barley, oats, and legumes—were cast aside; consumption of fatty meat increased. As a consequence, the composition of the average diet changed again. We began to eat more saturated fat, less fiber, and more easily digested carbohydrates. Something we didn't expect hap-pened, too—blood glucose after a meal became higher and more pro-longed, stimulating the pancreas to produce more insulin.

As a result of these developments, we not only experienced higher blood glucose levels after a meal, but we also experienced higher insulin responses. As we've mentioned, our bodies require insulin to metabolize carbohydrate, and insulin also has a profound effect on the development of many diseases. Researchers believe that high glucose and insulin lev-els are among the key factors responsible for heart disease and hyper-tension. And because insulin also influences the way we metabolize foods, it ultimately determines whether we store fat in our body.

Among the consequences of these major dietary changes, one is crucial for our discussion here: traditional diets all around the world contained slowly digested and absorbed carbohydrate—foods that we now know are low GI. On the other hand, our modern diet, with its rapidly digested carbohydrates, is based on high-GI foods. Thus, one of the most important ways in which our diet differs from that of our ancestors is the speed of carbohydrate digestion and the resulting effect on our blood glucose and insulin levels.

Insulin Plays Several Critical Roles in Our Health and Well-Being

ONE IMPORTANT FUNCTION of the **pancreas**, a vital organ near the stomach, is to produce the hormone **insulin**. Insulin plays several critical roles in our health and well-being.

First, it regulates our blood glucose levels. When you eat a meal containing carbohydrate, your blood glucose level rises. This increase causes the pancreas to secrete insulin (unless you have type 1 diabetes; see "What Is Diabetes?" in chapter 7), which pushes the glucose out of the bloodstream and into the muscles and tissues, where it provides **energy** for you to carry out your regular tasks and activities. The movement of glucose out of the blood and into the body's cells (its muscles and tissues) is finely controlled by just the right amount of insulin to drop the glucose back to normal.

Second, insulin plays a key part in determining the fuel mix that we burn from minute to minute—and whether we burn fat or carbohydrate to meet our energy needs. It does this by switching muscle cells from fat-burning to carb-burning. The relative proportions of fat to carbohydrate in your body's fuel are dictated by the prevailing levels of insulin in your blood. If insulin levels are low, as they are when you wake up in the morning, then the fuel you burn is mainly fat. If insulin levels are high, as they are after you consume a high-carbohydrate meal, then the fuel you burn is mainly carbohydrate.

Carbohydrates stimulate the secretion of insulin more than any other component of food. When carbohydrates are slowly absorbed by our bodies—which is the case with low-GI foods—the pancreas doesn't have to work as hard and produces less insulin. If the pancreas is overstimulated over a long period of time, which often occurs as a result of a diet rich in high-GI foods, it may become "exhausted," and type 2 diabetes may develop in genetically susceptible individuals. Even without diabetes, high insulin levels increase the risk of heart disease.

■ What We Eat Now ■

Today's western diet is the product of industrialization's many inventions—pasteurization, sterilization, refrigeration, freezing, roller drying, and spray drying, to name just a few. In the cereal-foods world, there's high-speed roller milling, high-temperature and high-pressure extrusion (think cereal flakes), puffing guns, short-time fermentation—you name it, they've invented it.

The benefits are many: we have a plentiful, relatively cheap, palatable (some would say too palatable!), and reasonably safe food supply. Gone are the days of monotonous meals, food shortages, and weevil-infested and otherwise spoiled food. Also long gone are such widespread vitamin deficiencies as scurvy and pellagra. Today's food manufacturers develop and sell delicious and safe products that satisfy just about everyone: foodies, the most health-conscious, and everyday supermarket shoppers alike.

Many of today's foods are still based on our original staples—wheat, corn, and oats—but the original grain has been ground down to produce fine flours with a small particle size that produce fine-quality breads, cakes, cookies, crackers, pastries, breakfast cereals, and snack foods. Cereal chemists and bakers know that the finest-particle-size flour produces the most palatable and shelf-stable end product.

Unfortunately, this striving for excellence has resulted in an unforeseen problem. Our bodies quickly digest and absorb many of the carbohydrate foods we consume the most—think corn flakes, white bread, instant rice. The resulting effect on blood glucose levels has created a problem of epidemic proportions.

■ What about Fat? ■

We've placed quite a bit of emphasis on carbohydrates, but our health is also affected by another key component in food, which often goes hand in hand with carbohydrates: **fat**. Food manufacturers, bakers, and chefs know we love to eat fat. We love its creaminess and feel in the mouth, and find it easy to consume in excess. Fat makes meat more tender, vegetables and salads more palatable, and sweet foods even more desirable. And fat makes numerous carbohydrates even tastier: with a wave of the fat wand, bland high-carbohydrate foods like rice, potatoes, and oats are magically transformed into highly palatable, calorically dense foods such as fried rice, French fries, and high-fat granola. In fact, when you analyze it, much of our diet today is an undesirable but delicious combination of fat and high-GI carbohydrates.

However, it's not just the amount of fat we eat but the type of fat that can lead to health problems. Most of the fat we now eat comes in the form of heart-unhealthy **saturated** or **trans fat**. Unlike unsaturated oils, which are liquid at room temperature, saturated fats and trans fats are solid at room temperature and clog up our arteries, among other problems. Unfortunately, the fats used for baking and frying are often saturated fats, such as hydrogenated vegetable oil or shortening. And much of the fat in *fatty* meats and dairy products is also saturated. But the fat in fish, olive oil, canola oil, and oil made from other seeds, such as safflower and sunflower, is the heart-healthy **unsaturated** kind.

Over the past twenty years, most health authorities wanted people to reduce the amount of saturated fat they ate. Unfortunately, *all* fats were lumped together as bad—the message "reduce fat" was easier than "reduce saturated fat." Today, we know that this simplified message was counterproductive. People avoided even the most essential of fats, the highly **polyunsaturated**, long-chain fats such as *omega-3s* that are fundamental to human health. We also avoided fat because of its high calorie content and tendency to be overeaten—only to replace it with large quantities of high-GI carbs that have the same properties and tendency to be overeaten. We fooled ourselves into thinking that any low-fat diet—especially one formulated with the help of a sophisticated food industry—was automatically a healthy diet. *But it's not.*

■ It's Not Just the Calories ■
We Take In . . .

A crucial point: we need to *balance* our food intake with the rate our bodies use it—that is, to eat the amount of calories from food that our bodies need, but not more. Consuming more calories than we expend is a recipe for gaining weight and experiencing health problems. That balance, as many of us know, is as difficult to achieve as ever.

Why? It's extremely easy to overeat. Refined foods, convenience foods, and fast foods tend to lack fiber and conceal fat; as a result, we often overdose on calories long before we realize we're full. And it's even easier *not* to exercise: it takes longer to walk somewhere than it does to drive, and our schedules are often so full that making time for physical activity seems impossible. That means we burn even fewer calories than we should, even as we're eating more and more. The result: our calorie intake exceeds our energy needs on a regular basis, and we gain weight.

Despite what many would have you believe, the answer to weight maintenance is *not* dieting most of the time—that is, reducing your food intake to a low level that matches a low level of energy expenditure. That's a recipe for failure. According to the Centers for Disease Control and Prevention, more than 95 percent of people who diet do not successfully keep the weight off. Nutritionists and public health experts are beginning to appreciate that a healthy diet comes in many different forms that may differ greatly in terms of proportions of fat, protein, and carbohydrate. That means that finding a solution that works for you has never been easier or more viable. We encourage you to choose the types of foods that suit your lifestyle and cultural and ethnic origins best, as these are the ones you are most likely to stick with for life.

Coupling a healthy, flexible diet you can live with long-term with an active lifestyle is the single best way to stay healthy and fit. That doesn't mean spending an hour at the gym six days a week. Instead, it means grabbing the opportunity for physical activity however and wherever you can. It means using the stairs, taking a ten-minute walk at lunchtime, using a treadmill while you watch the news, reading on an exercise bike, working in the garden, walking to stores, parking an extra distance from the office, or taking the dog for a walk each night. We know you have heard all this before. So whatever works for you, *do it*. Even housework burns calories. All of these seemingly small bursts of activity accumulate to increase our calorie burning. You don't have to take exercise very strenuously—just do it regularly.

Is there just one healthy diet that all of us should be following, with a set proportion of fat, carbohydrate, and protein? In other words, does one size fit all?

To be honest, we don't know—but research does show us that it's highly likely that we can be flexible. That said, we know there are two fundamental principles in *all* healthy diets: the carbohydrates are slow-release and the fat is relatively unsaturated (even when the intake is high).

Remember, no diet plan will work in the long term if it eliminates your favorite foods, whether these are bread or potatoes, ice cream, or pasta. The next chapter begins to tell you how you can eat a balanced and healthy diet—one tailored to *your* tastes and *your* needs—without feeling deprived. Part 4, Your Guide to Low-GI Eating, shows how easy it is to make the switch to low-GI eating for lifelong health and well-being. You may be surprised at just how simple and enjoyable incorporating the GI into your meals can be.

• 4 •

Carbohydrates—
The Big Picture: What They Are,
Why We Need Them,
How We Digest Them

*C*arbohydrate is the most widely consumed substance in the world after water. One of three main **macronutrients** (protein and fat are the other two), carbohydrate is a vital source of energy found in all plants and foods—including fruit, vegetables, cereals, and grains. The simplest form of carbohydrate is **glucose**, which is:

▶ a universal fuel for our bodies
▶ the only fuel source for our brain, red blood cells, and a growing fetus
▶ the main source of energy for our muscles during strenuous exercise

Some foods contain large amounts of carbohydrate (cereals, potatoes, sweet potatoes, legumes, and corn, for instance), while others, such as string beans, broccoli, and salad greens, have very small amounts of carbohydrate. Breast milk, cow's milk, and milk products (but not cheese) contain carbohydrate in the form of milk sugar or **lactose**.

What Exactly Is Carbohydrate?

CARBOHYDRATE IS A part of food. Starch is a carbohydrate; so, too, are sugars and nearly all dietary fiber. Starches and sugars are nature's reserves created by energy from the sun, carbon dioxide, and water.

The simplest form of carbohydrate is a single-sugar molecule called a **monosaccharide** (mono meaning one, saccharide meaning sweet). **Glucose** is a monosaccharide that occurs in food (as glucose itself and as the building block of starch) and is the most common source of fuel for the cells of the human body. **Fructose** and **galactose** are also monosaccharides.

If two monosaccharides are joined together, the result is a **disaccharide** (di meaning two). **Sucrose**, or common table sugar, is a disaccharide, as is **lactose**, the sugar in milk, and **maltose**.

As the number of monosaccharides in the chain increases, the carbohydrate becomes less sweet. Maltodextrins are **oligosaccharides** (oligo meaning a few) that are five or six glucose residues long. They taste only a little sweet and are commonly used as a food ingredient.

Starches are long chains of sugar molecules joined together like the beads in a string of pearls. They are called **polysaccharides** (poly meaning many). Starches are not sweet-tasting at all.

Dietary fibers are large carbohydrate molecules containing many different sorts of monosaccharides. They are different from starches and sugars because they are not broken down by human digestive enzymes. Dietary fiber is not digested in the small intestine; it thus reaches the large intestine without changing its form. Once there, bacteria begin to ferment and break down the fibers. As we previously noted in "The Effect of Fiber on the Glycemic Index" (see page 25, in chapter 2), different fibers have different physical and chemical properties. **Soluble fibers** are those that can be dissolved in water; some soluble fibers are very thick and therefore slow the speed of digestion. **Insoluble fibers**, on the other hand, such as cellulose, are not soluble in water and do not directly affect the speed of digestion.

As we explained at the beginning of this book, not all carbohydrates are created equal; in fact, they can behave quite differently in our bodies, and the GI is how we describe this difference. When you switch to eating predominantly low-GI carbs, which slowly trickle glucose into your bloodstream, you help to keep your blood glucose on an even keel and your energy levels perfectly balanced, and you'll feel fuller for longer periods between meals.

Sugars Found in Food

Monosaccharides (single-sugar molecules)	Disaccharides (two single-sugar molecules)
glucose	maltose = glucose + glucose
fructose	sucrose = glucose + fructose
galactose	lactose = glucose + galactose

Just as a car runs on fuel (gasoline), your body uses fuel (the food you eat). The fuel your body burns is derived from a mixture of the macronutrients—protein, fat, carbohydrates, and alcohol—that you consume. If you want to function well, be healthy, and feel your best, you need to fill your fuel tank—your body—with the right amount and the right kind of fuel every day.

Your body burns these macronutrients in a specific order—its **fuel hierarchy**. Because your body has no place to store unused alcohol, it tops the list. Protein comes second, followed by carbohydrate; fat comes in last. In practice, your body's fuel is usually a mix—a combination of carbohydrate and fat, in varying proportions. After meals, it's predominantly carbohydrates, and between meals, it's mainly fat.

Your body's ability to burn all the fat you eat is critical to weight control. If fat burning is inhibited, fat stores gradually accumulate. Because of this, the relative proportions of fat to carbohydrate in your body's fuel are critical (as we discussed in "Insulin Plays Several Critical Roles in Our Health and Well-Being," on page 32 in the previous chapter).

■ The Sources of Carbohydrates ■

The carbohydrate in our diet come primarily from plant foods—cereal grains, fruits, vegetables, and legumes (dried beans, chickpeas and lentils). Milk and foods made from milk (yogurt and ice cream, for example) also contain carbohydrate in the form of milk sugar, or lactose. *Lactose* is the first carbohydrate we encounter as infants; human milk contains more lactose than the milk of any other mammal, and it accounts for nearly half the energy that an infant will use. Some foods contain a large amount of carbohydrate (cereals, potatoes, and legumes, for instance); other foods, such as carrots, broccoli, and salad vegetables, contain minute amounts. Some vegetables contain so little carbohydrate we can't measure their GI.

Foods that are high in carbohydrate include:

▶ **Cereal grains:** rice, wheat, oats, barley, rye, and anything made from them—bread, pasta, noodles, flour, breakfast cereal
▶ **Fruits:** apples, bananas, grapes, apricots, peaches, plums, cherries, pears, mango, kiwi
▶ **Starchy vegetables:** potatoes, sweet potatoes, sweet corn, yams
▶ **Legumes:** all dried beans (kidney, black, cannellini), lentils, chickpeas, split peas
▶ **Dairy products:** yogurt, ice cream

SOURCES OF CARBOHYDRATE

PERCENTAGE OF CARBOHYDRATE (grams per 100 grams of food)			
apple	12%	peas	8%
baked beans	11%	pear	12%
banana	21%	plum	6%
barley	61%	potato	15%
bread	47%	raisins	75%
cornflakes	85%	rice	79%
flour	73%	split peas	45%

PERCENTAGE OF CARBOHYDRATE (grams per 100 grams of food)			
grapes	15%	sugar	100%
ice cream	22%	sweet corn	16%
milk	5%	sweet potato	17%
oats	61%	tapioca	85%
orange	8%	water cracker	71%
pasta	70%	wheat biscuit	62%

■ Turning Food into Fuel ■

To be able to use the carbohydrate in foods, your body has to break them down into a form that it can absorb and our cells can use; that process is digestion. To illuminate exactly what happens when your body digests food, here's how your body digests a piece of bread:

1. When you chew the bread in your mouth, it combines with saliva. Amylase, an enzyme in saliva, chops up the long-chain starch molecules in the bread into smaller-chain ones, such as maltose and maltodextrins (see "What Exactly Is Carbohydrate?" one page 38 for the definitions of these various molecules).

2. When you swallow the bread, it lands in your stomach; there it gets pummeled and churned, much like clothes in a washing machine. Once your stomach has squished it around, it spits out the bread into your small intestine. If the bread has viscous fibers in it (like oats and flax) or is acidic (like sourdough), mixing takes longer and the stomach empties more slowly.

3. Once the bread is in your small intestine, an avalanche of digestive juices attack any remaining bits of starch and break them down into smaller and smaller chains of glucose. Scientists call this process "overkill"; your body's goal is to turn everything into glucose. Many starches are rapidly digested, while others are more resistant, and thus the process is slower. The starch that

is inside any whole grains in your bread will be protected from attack and take longer to be broken down to glucose.

If the mixture of food and enzymes is highly viscous or sticky, owing to the presence of viscous fiber, mixing slows down, and the enzymes and starch take longer to make contact. The products of starch digestion will also take longer to move toward the wall of the intestine, where the last steps in digestion take place.

4. At the intestinal wall, the short-chain starch products, together with the sugars in foods, are broken down by specific enzymes. The monosaccharides that finally result from starch and sugar digestion include glucose, fructose, and galactose. These are absorbed from the small intestine into the bloodstream, where they are available to the cells as a source of energy.

5. Within five to ten minutes after eating, glucose appears in the bloodstream. The rate at which it appears (i.e., in a big gush, or as just a little trickle), is determined by the rate of digestion, as well as the rate at which food is emptied from the stomach. Together, these factors influence the GI of the food.

■ Carbohydrate Is Brain Food ■

Carbohydrate is your brain's essential fuel source. Except during starvation, carbohydrate is the only source of fuel that your brain can use. Your brain is the most energy-demanding organ in your body, responsible for over half your obligatory energy requirements. Unlike muscle cells, which can burn either fat or carbohydrate, the brain does not have the metabolic machinery to burn fat. If you fast for twenty-four hours, or decide not to eat carbohydrates, your brain will initially rely on small stores of carbohydrate in your liver; but within hours, these are depleted, and the liver begins synthesizing glucose from noncarbohydrate sources, including your muscle tissue. It has only a limited ability to do this, however, and any shortfall in glucose availability has consequences for brain function.

The benefits of carbohydrate on mental performance are well documented. Medical research shows us that people's intellectual performance dramatically improves after they eat carbohydrate-rich foods (or a glucose load). In recent studies, subjects were tested on various measures of "intelligence," including word recall, maze learning, arithmetic, short-term memory, rapid information processing, and reasoning. All types of people—young people, college students, people with diabetes, healthy elderly people, and those with Alzheimer's disease—showed an improvement in mental ability after they ate a meal containing carbohydrates. Interestingly, research shows that low-GI carbohydrates enhance learning and memory more than high-GI carbs, probably because there is no rebound fall in blood glucose.

Too little glucose can have serious physical consequences, as well; for a complete discussion, see chapter 8, where we discuss hypoglycemia, which results from low blood glucose.

■ What's Wrong with a ■ Low-Carbohydrate Diet?

Low-carbohydrate diets are nothing new: a low-carb diet to lose weight was first published in 1864. Low-carb diets are either high in protein or high in fat. They cannot be anything else, because we have to get our energy from something (and alcohol, the only other macronutrient, won't keep you alive for long).

There are at least two variations of carbohydrate intake on a low-carbohydrate diet; we'll confine our discussion to those where the reduction of carbohydrate is significant. There are those that are very low in carbohydrate, containing less than 100 grams of carbohydrate per day, and others that are *extremely low,* with reductions to as little as 20 to 30 grams of carbohydrate per day (ketogenic diets). The latter is the case with the first phase or "kick start" of various popular diet books and is not recommended for people with diabetes.

Without enough carbohydrate in your diet you may experience:

▶ Muscle fatigue, causing moderate exercise to be an enormous effort
▶ Insufficient fiber intake and therefore constipation
▶ Headaches and tiredness due to low blood glucose levels
▶ Bad breath due to the breakdown products of fat (ketones)

A recent review of low-carb diets has concluded that they are safe and effective (in terms of weight loss) in the short term, but there are potential risks in the long term (longer than six months).

One major concern is the potential for high saturated fat intake and the repercussions from that intake. Even a single meal high in saturated fat can have an adverse effect on blood vessels by inhibiting **vasodilation**, the normal increase in the diameter of blood vessels that occurs after a meal. The long-term effect of a low-carb diet would be an increase in **LDL cholesterol**. Compounding this, there may be a low intake of plant foods, which are normally considered protective against disease. Folate, fiber, and calcium contents of very low carbohydrate diets do not meet the Reference Daily Intake (RDI), formerly called the Recommended Daily Allowance (RDA).

Low-carb diets may also be high in protein (although not all high-protein diets are very low in carbohydrate). In people with diabetes, higher long-term dietary protein loads (over six months) may accelerate decline in renal function and increase calcium loss in urine, predisposing to osteoporosis and kidney stones.

To ensure that blood glucose levels can be maintained between meals, our bodies draw on the glucose stored in the liver; that form of glucose is called **glycogen**. Supplies of glycogen are strictly limited and must be replenished from meal to meal. If your diet is low in carbohydrate, your glycogen stores will be low as well, and easily depleted.

Once your body has used up its glycogen stores, which occurs twelve to twenty-four hours after you begin a fast, it will start breaking down muscle protein to create glucose for your brain and nervous system to use. However, this process can't supply all of the brain's needs. When absolutely necessary, the brain will make use of **ketones**, a by-product of the breakdown of fat. The level of ketones in the blood rises as the fast continues. You can even smell the ketones on the breath; they smell a little like apple cider.

In people who are losing weight on a low-carb diet, the level of ketones in the blood rises markedly, and this state, called **ketosis**, is taken as a sign of success. But the brain is definitely not at its best using ketones, and one result is that mental judgment is impaired. In all likelihood, you'll have a headache and feel mentally sluggish. Since your muscle stores of glycogen will have been depleted, you'll also find strenuous exercise almost impossible, and you may tire easily.

Here's How Weight Loss Works on a Low-Carb Diet

THE INITIAL WEIGHT loss on a low-carb diet is rapid; within the first few days, a dieter may lose 4 to 7 pounds. That's an encouraging sign to anyone trying to lose weight. The trouble is that most of that weight loss isn't fat, but muscle glycogen and water.

When you're no longer eating carbohydrate in sufficient amounts, your body uses its small carbohydrate reserves (glycogen, which is stored glucose) to fuel muscle contraction (in other words, movement). One gram of carbohydrate in the form of muscle and liver glycogen binds 4 grams of water. So when you use up your total reserves of 500 grams of glycogen within the first few days, you also lose 2 kilograms of water, for a total loss of 2.5 kilograms, or 5.5 pounds—*none* of it fat. When you return to normal eating, your carbohydrate reserves will be rapidly replenished, along with the water—meaning you'll put some or all of the weight right back on.

People who have followed low-carb diets for any length of time often notice that the rate at which they're losing weight plateaus fairly quickly, and they begin to feel rather tired and lethargic. That's not surprising, because without carbohydrates, the muscles have little glycogen stored. Strenuous exercise requires both fat and carbohydrate. So, in the long term, these low-carbohydrate diets may discourage people from the physical-exercise patterns that will help them keep their weight under control.

Our advice: the best diet for weight control is one you can stick to for life, which includes your favorite foods, and which accommodates your cultural and ethnic heritage. This diet can vary somewhat in total carbohydrate, protein, and fat. Currently, more scientific evidence supports the use of higher-fiber, higher-carbohydrate, low-GI, low-fat diets for weight loss. But the bottom line is that the *type* of carbohydrate and the *type* of fat are critical. Choosing low-GI foods will not only promote weight control, but it will also reduce blood glucose after meals, increase satiety, and provide bulk and a rich supply of micronutrients.

Ketosis is a serious concern for pregnant women. The fetus can be harmed and its brain development impaired by high levels of ketones crossing from the mother's blood via the placenta. Because being over-weight is often a cause of infertility, women who are losing weight may get pregnant unexpectedly. One of the primary reasons we advocate a healthy low-GI diet for pregnant women is that there are absolutely no safety concerns for mother and baby. Indeed, there is some evidence that a low-GI diet will help the mother control excessive weight gain during pregnancy.

·5·

How Much Carbohydrate Do You Need?

*M*ost of the world's population eats a high-carb diet based on staples such as rice, corn, millet, and wheat-based foods, such as bread or noodles. In some African and Asian countries, carbohydrates may form as much as 70 to 80 percent of a person's caloric intake—though this is probably too high for optimum health. In contrast, most people in industrialized countries eat only half of these carbohydrate calories. Our diets typically contain about 40 to 45 percent carbohydrate and 33 to 40 percent fat.

▪ What Is the Optimal Level of ▪ Carbohydrates You Should Be Eating?

We believe your carbohydrate intake can be *either* moderate or high, but that the *type* and *source* of the carbohydrate and the fat that you eat are as important as the amount.

By high, we mean that more than 50 to 55 percent of your total daily calories is from carbs; by moderate, we mean that about 40 to 50 percent of total daily calories is from carbs.

If you look carefully at diets all around the world, it's clear that both high and moderate intakes of carbohydrate are commensurate with good health; the choice is ultimately up to you. Both types of diets, however, need to emphasize low-GI carbs and healthy fats. The way of eating that you'll enjoy and tend to follow over the long term is the one that is closest to your usual diet. Our approach has built-in flexibility when it comes to the amount of carbohydrate you need to eat.

In fall 2002 the National Institutes of Health (NIH) published new nutritional guidelines suggesting a range of carbohydrate intakes that could adequately meet the body's needs while minimizing your disease risk. We like the NIH's figures in part because they allow for individual tailoring. Specifically, they advised the following ranges:

- **Carbohydrate:** 45–65% of energy
- **Fat:** 25–35% of energy
- **Protein:** 15–35% of energy

Chances are your diet already falls within these flexible ranges; if so, we encourage you to stick with what you have. If your preference is for more protein and more fat than you are currently eating, then go ahead—just be choosy about the quality. (For more about protein, see "The Real Deal on Protein and Health," pages 50–51.) We believe that you are the best judge of what you can live with. However, we do recommend that you consume at least 130 grams of carbohydrate a day, even if you are on a weight-loss program. Whatever the number, the type of carbohydrate is important, and that's where the GI comes to the fore.

How to Find a Dietitian

FOR SPECIFIC INFORMATION about your own calorie and exact carbohydrate needs, you should consult a registered dietitian (RD). Your primary care physician or a medical specialist you see for a specific condition may have one or more dietitians in their practice. Alternatively, look in the Yellow Pages under Dietitians, call the American Dietetic Association's Consumer Nutrition Hotline (800-366-1655), or go to the ADA's home page: www.eatright.org. Make sure that the person you choose has the letters RD after his or her name.

■ Is a High-Carbohydrate ■ Diet for You?

Is consuming 50 percent or more of your calories from carbohydrates and less than 30 percent from fats (the remaining 15 percent or more should come from protein) realistic for you? That depends. If you have always been health conscious and avoided high-fat foods, or if you follow an Asian or Middle Eastern diet, then chances are you're already eating a high-carbohydrate diet, and it's a good choice for you.

Of course, the number of calories and the amount of carbohydrate varies with your weight and activity levels. If you're an active person—as we hope you are—with average energy requirements who is not trying to lose weight (i.e., with an average intake of 2,000 calories per day), you will require 275 grams of carbohydrate. If you are trying to lose weight and are consuming a low-calorie diet (in other words, you're a small eater on 1,200 calories per day), that means you should be eating about 165 grams of carbohydrate a day. As an example of what these diets look like, see pages 55 to 58.

■ Is a Moderate Carbohydrate ■ Diet for You?

North Americans tend to eat too many calories from all food sources. The reason: typical American portions of carbohydrate and protein are oversized (and should be reduced). A Mediterranean-type diet is higher in fat and provides about 45 to 50 percent of energy as carbohydrate. In the past, most nutritionists would have frowned upon this, but that's no longer the case, as research has shown that this type of diet can have important health benefits. As long as you carefully consider the types of fat and the types of carbohydrate you're eating, then this level of carbohydrate intake is perfectly commensurate with good health. At this level, you need to consume at least 130 grams of carbohydrate a day if you are a small eater and 225 grams if you are an average eater. See page 216, for an idea of how many servings of bread, cereal, pasta, or rice will provide these amounts of carbohydrate.

The Real Deal on Protein and Health

ADDING MORE PROTEIN to your diet makes good sense for weight control. In comparison with carbohydrate and fat, protein makes us feel more satisfied immediately after eating it and reduces hunger between meals. In addition, protein increases our metabolic rate for one to three hours after eating. This means we burn more energy by the minute compared with the increase that occurs after eating carbs or fats. Protein foods are also excellent sources of micronutrients, such as iron, zinc, vitamin B_{12}, and omega-3 fats.

Which foods are high in protein?

The best sources of protein are meats (beef, pork, lamb, chicken), fish, and shellfish. As long as these are trimmed of fat and not served with creamy sauces, you can basically eat to suit your appetite, though you'll find your appetite for lean protein will have a natural limit. When buying protein foods, choose the leanest cuts, remove all the visible fat, and grill, bake, braise, stir-fry, or pan-sauté.

Another excellent source of protein is legumes—a low-GI food that is easy on the budget, versatile, filling, nutritious, and low in calories. Legumes are high in fiber, too—both soluble and insoluble—and are packed with nutrients, providing a valuable source (in addition to protein) of carbohydrate, B vitamins, iron, zinc, magnesium, and phytochemicals (natural plant chemicals that possess antiviral, antifungal, antibacterial, and anticancer properties). Whether you buy dried beans, lentils, and chickpeas and cook them yourself at home, or opt for the very convenient, time-saving canned varieties, you are choosing one of nature's lowest-GI foods.

Dairy products are also good sources of protein—and the combination of protein and calcium that is unique to dairy foods can aid weight control. Research has shown that the more calcium or dairy foods (it's hard to separate the two) people eat, the lower their weight and fat mass. Calcium is intimately involved in burning fat—a process we want to encourage. Choose low-fat dairy products, including milk, yogurt, and cottage cheese. Go easy on high-fat cheeses such as cheddar, feta, Camembert, and Brie—though you don't have to cut them out entirely. It's better to have a small serving of one of these cheeses than a giant serving of a reduced-fat version that doesn't taste anywhere near as good.

Nuts are excellent sources of protein, dietary fiber, and micronutrients—and they contain very little saturated fat (the fats are predominantly mono- or polyunsaturated). With nuts, take care not to overeat them, because they're **energy dense**—meaning they pack a lot of calories into a small weight. Research suggests that eating a small handful of nuts (1 ounce) several times a week can help lower cholesterol and reduce heart attack risk. If you eat them as a snack, put a small handful in a small bowl; don't eat them straight from the package. (See page 193 for more recommendations about eating nuts.)

For a number of years now, eggs have been shedding their undeservedly bad reputation brought on because of their cholesterol content; in fact, they are a great source of protein and several essential vitamins and minerals. We now know that high blood cholesterol results from eating large amounts of saturated fat (rather than cholesterol) in foods. And if you select omega-3-enriched eggs, you will increase your intake of good fat as well as your protein intake.

Can you eat too much protein?

The American Institute of Medicine recommends that no more than 35 percent of energy in our diets come from protein. That is, 175 grams of pure protein for a person consuming 2,000 calories a day. In practice, most people will have no desire to eat beyond that amount.

A high-protein intake has been criticized because it might also mean a high intake of saturated fat—which shouldn't happen if you stick to lean meat and low-fat dairy products. Concerns about the effect of high protein intake on kidney function are limited to people who already have compromised kidney function—some people with diabetes, the very elderly, and infants.

■

**When you eat low-GI carbs, your insulin levels will
be lower and you will automatically burn more fat.
You may not feel this change as it is happening, but
you will see the results—you'll lose weight—over
time. Eating high-fiber foods will also help fill you
up and keep you from overeating.**

■

■ The Best Ways to Eat Carbs ■

To ensure that you are eating enough carbs, and the right kind of carbohydrate, you should eat:

- fruits at every meal
- vegetables with lunch and dinner and even as snacks
- at least one low-GI food at each meal
- at least the minimum quantity of carbohydrate foods suggested for small eaters (see pages 55–56)
- lots of fiber (bulky foods with low energy density, or fewer calories per gram)

If you are looking for ways to improve your own diet, here are two important things for you to remember:

- Identify the sources of carbohydrate in your diet and reduce high-GI foods. Don't go to extremes; there is room for your favorite high-GI foods.
- Identify the sources of fat and look at ways you can reduce saturated fat. Choose monounsaturated and polyunsaturated fats, such as olive oil and sunflower oil, instead of saturated fats like butter and shortening. Again, don't go overboard—the body needs some fat, and there's room for your favorite fatty foods on occasion. Just remember to watch your portions.

■

To determine the percentage of calories you get from carbohydrate in a food, multiply the grams of carbohydrate by 4 (the number of calories supplied per gram of carbohydrate) and then divide by the total number of calories.

For example, take a container of yogurt with 25 grams of carbohydrate:

$$25 \times 4 \div 180 = 55\%$$
of calories from carbohydrate

■

■ The Right Kind of Carbohydrate Diet for You ■

To help guide your daily food choices, we've created two GI food pyramids, one for high-carbohydrate eaters, the other for moderate-carbohydrate eaters. (If you're a big bread and cereal eater, the GI pyramid for high-carb eaters will suit you better.) The recommended servings of each food group are shown within each pyramid. In either case, "How Much Is a Serving?" below, applies to both pyramids.

If you're pregnant or breast-feeding or are interested in more detailed nutrition guidelines for your children, talk to your dietitian or doctor (see "How to Find a Dietitian," page 48), or visit www.health ierus.gov/dietaryguidelines/. For further guidance about children and the GI, see chapter 11.

■ How Much Is a Serving? ■

Whether you eat carbs in moderate or large amounts, the portion sizes stay the same.

Indulgences
2 tablespoons cream, sour cream
1 ounce chocolate
1 small slice (about 1½ ounces) cake

1 small bag (1 ounce) potato chips
2 standard alcoholic drinks (a 5-ounce glass of wine, 1½ ounces of distilled spirits, or a 12-ounce beer)

Fish, seafood, lean meats, poultry, eggs, and alternatives
3 ounces (cooked) boneless meat, fish, or chicken
3 ounces canned fish
2 eggs
1½ ounces reduced-fat cheese or 1 ounce full-fat cheese
3½ ounces tofu

Legumes
½ cup cooked lentils, chickpeas, or beans

Low-fat dairy or alternative
1 cup milk or soy milk
1 cup yogurt

Nuts and oils
2 teaspoons olive or canola oil
1 tablespoon oil-based vinaigrette
½ ounce nuts
¼ cup avocado

Breads, cereals, rice, pasta, noodles, and grains
1 slice bread
½ cup cooked rice, pasta, or noodles
½ cup cereal

Fruit and juices
1 medium piece of fruit
1 cup small fruit pieces
½ cup juice

Vegetables
½ cup cooked vegetables
1 cup raw or salad vegetables

The Glycemic Index Pyramid for **HIGH**-Carbohydrate Eaters

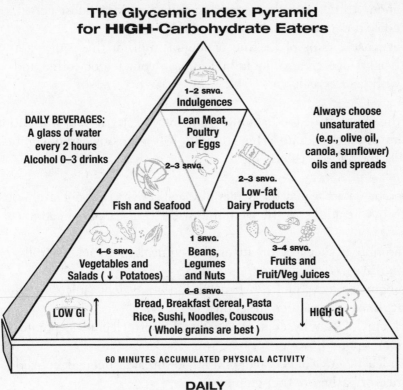

DAILY BEVERAGES:
A glass of water
every 2 hours
Alcohol 0–3 drinks

1–2 SRVG.
Indulgences

**Lean Meat,
Poultry
or Eggs**

Always choose
unsaturated
(e.g., olive oil,
canola, sunflower)
oils and spreads

2–3 SRVG.

Fish and Seafood

2–3 SRVG.
**Low-fat
Dairy Products**

4–6 SRVG.
**Vegetables and
Salads (↓ Potatoes)**

1 SRVG.
**Beans,
Legumes
and Nuts**

3–4 SRVG.
**Fruits and
Fruit/Veg Juices**

6–8 SRVG.

LOW GI ↑

**Bread, Breakfast Cereal, Pasta
Rice, Sushi, Noodles, Couscous
(Whole grains are best)**

HIGH GI ↓

60 MINUTES ACCUMULATED PHYSICAL ACTIVITY

DAILY

■ A High-Carbohydrate Diet ■

Below is an example of what's involved in eating a high-carbohydrate diet
(65% of total daily energy from carbohydrates) for small or average eaters.

Small eaters ■ may be small-framed females ■ have small appetites
■ do very little physical activity ■ be trying to lose weight. Even the
smallest eater needs carbohydrate-rich foods like the ones described
below every day:

- around 4 slices of bread or the equivalent (crackers, rolls,
  English muffins)
- at least 2 pieces of fresh fruit or the equivalent (juice, dried
  fruit, or fruit canned in its own juice)
- about 1 cup of starchy cooked vegetables (corn, legumes,
  potato, sweet potato)

- about 1 cup of cooked cereal or grain food (breakfast cereal, cooked rice or pasta, or other grains)
- at least 2 cups of fat-free or low-fat milk or the equivalent (yogurt, ice cream), including milk in your tea or coffee and with your cereal

If this amount of food sounds right for you, try it as a minimum amount of carbohydrate. This supplies 190 grams of carbohydrates, suitable for a 1,200-calorie diet.

Average eaters ■ may do regular physical activity (but not strenuous exercise) ■ be adults of average frame size. Average eaters need to eat:

- around 8 slices of bread or the equivalent (crackers, rolls, muffins)
- about 4 pieces of fresh fruit or the equivalent (juice, dried fruit, or fruit canned in its own juice)
- 1 cup of starchy cooked vegetables (corn, legumes, potato, sweet potato)
- at least 2 cups of cereal or grain food (breakfast cereal, cooked rice or pasta, or other grains)
- 2 cups of low-fat milk or the equivalent (yogurt, ice cream)

This provides 250 grams of carbohydrate, which is suitable for an 1,800-calorie diet.

Overeating is highly unlikely on the high-fiber, high-carbohydrate, low-fat diet described above, because these foods tend to be so filling and satisfying. So base your diet on high-fiber carbohydrate foods like whole-grain breads, cereals, fruit, vegetables, and legumes, and let your appetite dictate how much you need to eat.

■ A Moderate-Carbohydrate Diet ■

If you think you'd prefer a more moderate carbohydrate intake (45 percent of total daily energy) and more fat, then here's an example of how much carbohydrate small and average eaters would need each day.

The Glycemic Index Pyramid for **MODERATE**-Carbohydrate Eaters

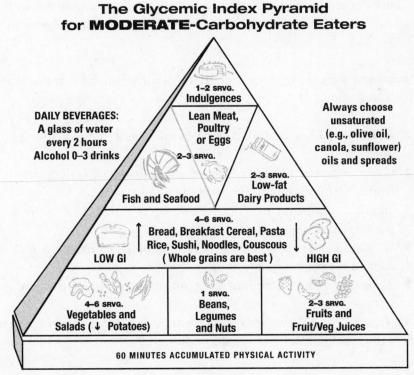

DAILY BEVERAGES:
A glass of water every 2 hours
Alcohol 0–3 drinks

Always choose unsaturated (e.g., olive oil, canola, sunflower) oils and spreads

1–2 SRVG. **Indulgences**

Lean Meat, Poultry or Eggs
2–3 SRVG.

Fish and Seafood

2–3 SRVG. **Low-fat Dairy Products**

4–6 SRVG. **Bread, Breakfast Cereal, Pasta Rice, Sushi, Noodles, Couscous** (Whole grains are best)
LOW GI   HIGH GI

4–6 SRVG. **Vegetables and Salads (↓ Potatoes)**

1 SRVG. **Beans, Legumes and Nuts**

2–3 SRVG. **Fruits and Fruit/Veg Juices**

60 MINUTES ACCUMULATED PHYSICAL ACTIVITY

DAILY

Small eaters: For a balanced intake of nutrients on a moderate-carbohydrate diet, even a small eater needs these carbohydrate foods every day:

▶ around 4 slices of bread or the equivalent (crackers, rolls, English muffins)
▶ at least 2 pieces of fresh fruit or the equivalent (juice, dried fruit, or fruit canned in its own juice)

- about ½ cup of cooked starchy vegetables (corn, legumes, potato, sweet potato)
- about ½ cup of cereal or grain food (breakfast cereal, cooked rice or pasta, or other grains)
- 2 cups of low-fat milk or the equivalent (yogurt, ice cream)

These carbohydrate foods supply 135 grams of carbohydrate, which is about 45 percent of total daily energy from carbohydrates in a 1,200-calorie diet.

Average eaters: Even on a moderate-carbohydrate diet, the average eater needs to eat:

- around 6 slices of bread or the equivalent (crackers, rolls, muffins)
- about 2 pieces of fresh fruit or the equivalent (juice, dried fruit, or fruit canned in its own juice)
- about ½ cup of high-carbohydrate vegetables (corn, legumes, potato, sweet potato)
- at least 1½ cups of cereal or grain food (breakfast cereal, cooked rice or pasta, or other grain)
- 2½ cups of low-fat milk or the equivalent (yogurt, ice cream)

This provides 200 grams of carbohydrates, which is 45 percent of total daily energy in an 1,800-calorie diet.

■ How to Switch to a Lower-GI Diet Today ■

Readers and our clients report that the following foods are those they began eating in order to achieve a low-GI diet:

- grainy breads
- low-GI breakfast cereals
- more fruit
- yogurt
- pasta

- legumes
- vegetables

In part 4, Your Guide to Low-GI Eating, we give you many ways to make the change to a low-GI diet (see chapter 14), along with the low-GI food finder, pantry planner, cooking tips, and more than 45 fast, delicious recipes making the most of low-GI ingredients.

PART 2

The Glycemic Index and Your Health

How the glycemic index can help you with weight control, diabetes, hypoglycemia, heart health, the metabolic syndrome (insulin resistance syndrome, formerly known as syndrome X), and polycystic ovarian syndrome (PCOS)—as well as how children and athletes can use the GI.

· 6 ·

The Glycemic Index
and Weight Control

*O*besity **is a** serious and growing health threat for a large percentage of North America's population. Between 1991 and 2000,
obesity in the United States rose 60 percent, and today, two out of
three American adults are overweight and one in three is obese. Even
children are at risk; over 19 percent of American children are **overweight**, and the number is growing by the day. Although obesity rates
for both adults and children are significantly lower in Canada (see box
on page 64), it's a large and growing problem there, too, along with the
health issues that accompany it. There is no simple solution to this epidemic. The problem needs to be tackled on many fronts, including
exercise and diet. We do know that the glycemic index is a practical
tool in the nutrition toolbox—one that plays an important role in
weight management by helping to control appetite and insulin levels.

If you're overweight, chances are that you've read countless books,
brochures, and magazines that offer "diet plans" and quick-fix ways to
slim down. But for the majority of people who are overweight, these
methods don't work—if they did, there wouldn't be so many still on
the market.

Obesity Rates in the United States versus Canada

OVER THE PAST decade, Canada's obesity rates have been based on self-reported data, whereas the United States has derived rates from actual measurements of height and weight since the early 1960s. With the measured data from the 2004 Canadian Community Health Survey, it is possible to compare the current prevalence of obesity in the two countries.

Age-standardized results show that 30 percent of Americans age eighteen or older were obese in 1999–2002, significantly above the Canadian rate of 23 percent. Most of this difference was attributable to the situation among women. While 23 percent of Canadian women were obese, the figure for American women was 33 percent.

That's because at best a diet will help you reduce your calorie intake, at least as long as you're sticking to it, which may bring some weight loss. At its worst, a diet will change your body composition for the fatter. That's because many diets employ the technique of drastically reducing your carbohydrate intake to bring about quick weight loss. The weight you lose, however, is mostly water (that was trapped or held with stored carbohydrate) and muscle (as it is broken down to produce the glucose you need to fuel your brain). Once you return to your former way of eating, your body contains a little less muscle mass. But because muscle mass burns significantly more calories than fat, you need even less food than you did before you started dieting—which means you're more likely to put on weight.

Thus begins the yo-yo weight gain, weight loss pattern that is all too familiar to so many dieters. The overall effect of this pattern is a weight increase of from four to seven pounds a year. Why? When you lose weight through severely restricting your food intake, you lose some of your body's muscle mass. Over the years, yo-yo dieting changes your body's composition to less muscle and proportionately more fat, making weight control increasingly more difficult. Your body's engine requires less and less fuel to keep it running.

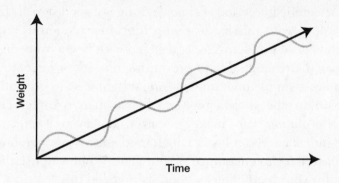

FIGURE 7. The yo-yo effect of restrictive dieting

That's why we're not prescribing yet another diet for you to try. Instead, our focus is on presenting important facts about food and how your body uses it. Because not all foods are equal, when it comes to losing weight, it's not necessarily a matter of reducing how much you eat, but rather, changing the types of foods you choose. Research has shown that the type of food you give your body determines what it is going to burn and what it is going to store as body fat. Studies also show that certain foods are more satisfying to the appetite than others.

This is where the glycemic index plays a leading role. Low-GI foods have two essential advantages for people trying to lose weight:

▶ They fill you up and keep you satisfied longer.
▶ They help you burn more body fat and less muscle.

Eating to lose weight with low-GI foods is easier because you don't have to go hungry—so you won't overeat or make poor food choices because you're ravenous—and what you end up with is true fat loss, rather than water or muscle loss.

■ Being Overweight Puts You at Increased Risk ■

As you may know, being overweight puts you at an increased risk for a range of health problems. Among these are heart disease, diabetes, high blood pressure, gout, gallstones, sleep apnea (when breathing stops for a significant period of time; snoring is a good sign of this), and arthritis. Along with this list of **complications**, numerous emotional and psychological problems are associated with being overweight.

It's clear that the answer to preventing obesity or becoming over-weight is not a simple one, nor is losing weight easy to do—otherwise weight wouldn't be such a problem for so many people. *The New Glucose Revolution* can make it easier, however. Thanks to the glycemic index, we can tell you which foods satisfy hunger longer and are the least likely to encourage weight gain. When you use the GI as the basis for your food choices, there is no need to:

▶ overly restrict your food intake
▶ obsessively count calories
▶ starve yourself

Learning which foods your body works best on is what using the glycemic index is all about.

It is also worthwhile to take control of aspects of your life that have an impact on your weight. You may not create a new body from your efforts, but you will feel better about the body you've got. Eating well and exercising is the aim of the game.

■ Why Do People Become Overweight? ■

Is it genetic? Is it hormonal? Is it our environment? Is it a psycholog-ical problem? Or is it due to an abnormal metabolism?

For a few blessed individuals, a constant weight is maintained year in and year out without much conscious effort. Often, these people are naturally active and their body instinctively gravitates to a healthy weight. For others, who are overweight, regardless of all their efforts to control it—every fad diet, every exercise program, even medications and weight-loss operations—body weight is eventually regained. Why?

Our weight is a result of how much we take in and how much we burn. So, if we take in too much and don't burn enough, we are like-ly to put on weight. The question is, then: how much, and of what, is too much?

The answer is not a simple one: not all foods are equal, and no two bodies are the same.

People are overweight for many different reasons. Research shows us that a combination of social, genetic, dietary, metabolic, psychological, and emotional factors combine to influence our weight.

First, let's look at the role genetics plays in weight control. There are many overweight people who tell us resignedly: "Well, my mother's/father's the same," or "I've always been overweight," or "It must be in my genes."

These comments have much truth behind them. A child born to overweight parents is much more likely to be overweight than one whose parents are not overweight. It may sound like an excuse, but there is a lot of evidence to back up the idea that our body weight and shape is at least partially determined by our genes.

Much of our knowledge in this area comes from studies of twins. Identical twins tend to be similar in body weight even if they are raised apart. Twins adopted as infants show the body-fat profile of their biological parents rather than that of their adoptive parents. In one study, when twins were given 1,000 extra calories a day for 100 days, some gained 9 pounds and some gained 26 pounds, but amazingly, one twin invariably gained similar amounts to that of his/her twin. These findings suggest that our genes are a stronger determinant of weight than our environment (which includes the food we eat). It seems that information stored in our genes governs our tendency to burn off or store excess calories.

Our genetic makeup also underlies our **metabolism** (basically, how many calories we burn per minute). Bodies, like cars, differ in this regard. A V-8 engine consumes more fuel to run than a small car with a four-cylinder engine. A bigger body generally requires more calories than a smaller one. When a car is stationary, the engine idles—using just enough fuel to keep the motor running. When we are asleep, our engine keeps running (for example, our brain is still at work) and we use a minimum number of calories. This is our *resting metabolic rate*—the amount of calories we burn without any exercise (when we are at rest). Most of it is necessary fuel for our large brains. When we start exercising, or even just moving around, the number of calories, or the amount of fuel we use, increases. The largest amount (around 70 percent) of the calories used in a twenty-four-hour period, however, those used to maintain our resting metabolic rate.

Since our resting metabolic rate accounts for how most of the calories we eat are used, it is a significant determinant of our body weight. The lower your resting metabolic rate, the greater your risk of gaining weight and vice versa. We all know someone who appears to eat all the time but manages to stay reed thin. Almost in awe (or with envy) we comment on their "fast metabolism"—and we may not be far off the mark. Whether you have a low or high resting metabolic rate is genetically determined.

How much muscle you have affects your resting metabolic rate, too. Men have a higher resting metabolic rate than women, because their bodies contain more muscle mass and are more expensive to run; body fat, on the other hand, gets a free ride. These days, too many men and women have undersized muscles that hardly ever get a workout. Increasing muscle mass with weight-bearing (resistance) exercise will raise your resting metabolic rate and is one of the secrets to lifelong weight control.

Calories—Measuring the Fuel You Need

CALORIES ARE A measure of the energy in food and the energy you require to keep you alive. Your body needs a certain number of calories every day to keep your heart beating and your brain working. Food and drink are the source of calories, and if you eat and drink too much, you store the additional calories as extra body fat and protein. If you consume fewer calories than you need, your body will break down its stores of fat and protein—which leads to weight loss—to make up for the shortage

The calorie content of a food is often considered a measure of how fattening it is. Carbohydrate and protein yield the fewest calories per gram; fat, the highest, as follows:

carbohydrate	4 calories per gram
protein	4 calories per gram
alcohol	7 calories per gram
fat	9 calories per gram

Our genes also dictate the fuel mix we burn in the fasting state (overnight). Some of us burn more carbohydrate and less fat even though the total energy used (calories burned) is the same. Scientists believe that subtle abnormalities in the ability to burn fat (as opposed to carbohydrate) lie behind most states of being overweight and obese.

All this doesn't mean that if your parents were overweight you should resign yourself to being overweight, too. But it may help you understand why you have to watch what you eat while other people seemingly don't have to. One way in which *The New Glucose Revolution* helps is that it facilitates greater use of fat as a source of fuel.

So if you were born with a tendency to be overweight, why does it matter what you eat? The answer is that foods are not equal in their effect on body metabolism. In particular, the foods you eat dictate the fuel mix that you burn for several hours after eating. If you're burning more fat and less carbohydrate, even if the energy content of the food is the same, then chances are you'll be less hungry and less likely to gain body fat over the course of the day. (See "Insulin Plays Several Critical Roles in Our Health and Well-Being" in chapter 3.)

Consequently, your choice of foods is critical for weight control. In fact, by being choosy about carbohydrates and fats, you maximize **insulin sensitivity** (see more about this on page 118 in chapter 7), turn "up" the genes involved in burning fat, and turn "down" those involved in burning carbs. By moving your fuel currency exchange from a carbohydrate economy to a fat economy, you increase the opportunity to deplete fat stores over carbohydrate stores. This is exactly what will happen when you begin to eat low-GI foods.

■ Fine-Tuning the Message ■
About Diets for Weight Control

Among all four major sources of calories in food (protein, fat, carbohydrate, and alcohol), fat has the highest energy content per gram, twice that of carbohydrate and protein (see "Calories—Measuring the Fuel You Need" on page 68). A high-fat food is therefore said to be *energy dense*, meaning there are a lot of calories in a relatively small amount of food. A typical croissant made with wafer-thin layers of buttery pastry contains about 500 calories (which equals about 20–25 percent of most people's total energy needs for the day). To eat the same amount of energy (calories) in the form of apples, you have to eat about six large apples. So eating energy-dense foods makes it all too easy to get more calories than your body needs.

Energy Density—Key Things to Know

A FOOD'S **ENERGY DENSITY**—the number of calories per gram or per serving size—is more important to weight control than its fat content. Some diets, such as traditional Mediterranean diets, contain quite a lot of fat (mainly from olive oil) but are still bulky—meaning they're filling without being high in calories. This is because they are based on large portions of fruits and vegetables, including foods like legumes, and they also have exceptionally low GI values. These diets consequently have a lower overall energy density.

Many new low-fat foods on the market are not bulky—they have the same energy density, or amount of calories, as the original high-fat food. Examples include low-fat yogurts, ice creams, and sweet and savory snack products. So read the label—look for the energy (calorie) content per 100 grams or per serving as your best guide to a food's "fattening" power—recognizing that fewer than 120 calories per 100 grams qualifies it as having low energy density.

You can eat quantity—just consider the quality of what you're eating!

During the 1990s, one of the most notable research findings within the nutrition community was that high-fat foods were less satiating than conventional high-carbohydrate foods. For this reason, experts advised dieters to stay away from high-fat foods, and the food industry developed and flooded the market with more low-fat foods. Unfortunately, along the way, someone forgot to say that what *really* counts is a food's final energy density—the total amount of calories it contains. If a low-fat food has the same energy density as a high-fat food, then it's just as easy to overconsume. Lots of low-fat products on the market are no different from their high-fat counterparts when it comes to calories per gram (think low-fat yogurts, ice cream, crackers, and cookies).

Nutritionists have therefore had to fine-tune the message about diets for weight control:

▶ Eating more fruits and vegetables is more important than simply eating less fat.
▶ The type of fat is more critical than the amount.
▶ The type of carbohydrate is important, too.

A GI Success Story

"I'VE NEVER BEEN thin, but after the birth of my last child, I weighed in at over 270 pounds. Not surprisingly, I was miserable, and I constantly felt sick. So I decided it was time to make a change. I began eating a high-carbohydrate, low-GI diet (I hesitate to even call it a diet, because diets fail, and this one didn't!) and started exercising more often. Within a year, I'd lost 100 pounds! But just as important, I felt—and feel—so much better. I have tons of energy, and I no longer suffer from acid reflux; even my skin looks great. I've never been healthier in my life."

—Jeanne

■ Exactly Why Exercise Is ■ So Beneficial for Weight Control

Exercise doesn't just burn calories while you're doing it: people who exercise have higher metabolic rates and their bodies burn more calories per minute all day long, even when they're asleep.

A fast metabolism is not always a matter of genetic "luck." Exercise, or any physical activity, speeds up our metabolic rate. By increasing our energy (caloric) expenditure, exercise helps to balance our energy (calorie) intake from food.

Exercise also builds muscle, and bigger muscles demand more energy and are better at using the fat in your body as fuel. Plus, by making your muscles more sensitive to insulin, exercise reduces the body's demand for insulin and increases the amount of fat you burn. A low-GI diet has the same effect. Low-GI foods reduce the amount of insulin you need, which makes fat easier to burn and harder to store. When you eat a low-GI meal, the fuel mix being burned for the next few hours contains more fat and less carbohydrate. Since body fat is what you want to get rid of when you lose weight, exercise in combination with a low-GI diet makes a lot of sense.

Notably, a team of Austrian researchers led by Dr. Babak Bahadori reported in the journal *Diabetes, Obesity and Metabolism* (July 2005) that a low-fat, low-GI diet actually reduced the amount of muscle loss—but not the amount of fat loss—that people experienced when attempting to lose weight. This is especially important because muscle burns up to thirty times the amount of calories per pound that fat does, so it's crucial for keeping your metabolism revved and your weight in check.

■

Your goal when losing weight should be to lose fat, not muscle or water weight.

■

■ Energy-Dense Foods—Not Sugary and Starchy ■ Foods—Most Affect Your Weight

For many years it was widely—and wrongly—believed that sugar and starchy foods like potatoes, rice, and pasta were the cause of obesity. Twenty-five years ago, every weight-loss diet advocated restriction of these carbohydrate-rich foods. One reason stemmed from the "instant" results of low-carbohydrate diets. As we mentioned above, if your diet is very low in carbohydrate, you will lose weight fast—but that lost weight is all fluid and often muscle rather than fat. Moreover, a low-carbohydrate diet depletes the limited carbohydrate (glycogen) stores in the muscles, making exercise difficult and tiring.

Sugar, too, has been blamed for obesity, because it is often found in such energy-dense foods as cakes, cookies, chocolate, and ice cream. These foods, however, contain a mixture of sugar and fat—and it's the fat that makes them so high in calories. The reality is that the primary sources of calories (concentrated energy) in most people's diets are not sweet. Instead, they're often fatty meats, cheese, French fries, potato chips, rich sauces, crackers, butter, and margarine—foods that contain no sugar at all.

On the whole, there is scant evidence to condemn sugar or starchy foods as the cause of obesity. Overweight people show a preference for high-calorie foods rather than a preference for foods high in sugar or starch, because their bodies have high energy requirements, even at rest, and the easiest way to satisfy their hunger is with high-energy foods. In a survey conducted at the University of Michigan in which obese men and women listed their favorite foods, men preferred mainly fatty meats, and women listed cakes, cookies, and doughnuts. The unifying trait was a lot of energy per gram of food.

■ How the Glycemic Index ■ Helps You Lose Weight

One of the biggest challenges to losing weight can be feeling hungry all the time, but this gnawing feeling is not a necessary part of losing weight. Foods with low GI values are among the most filling of all foods and delay hunger pangs longer. To date, more than twenty studies around the world have confirmed the remarkable fact that low-GI foods, in comparison with their nutrient-matched high-GI counterparts, are more filling, delay hunger pangs longer, and/or reduce energy intake for the remainder of the day.

In the past, it was believed that protein, fat, and carbohydrate foods, taken in equal quantities, satisfied our appetite equally. We now know from recent research that the *satiating capacity*—the degree to which foods make us feel full—of these three nutrients is not equal.

Fatty foods, in particular, have only a weak effect on satisfying appetite relative to the number of calories they provide. This has been demonstrated clearly in experimental situations in which people are asked to eat until their appetite is satisfied. They overconsume calories if the foods they are offered are high in fat. When high-carbohydrate and low-fat foods are offered, they consume fewer calories when given the opportunity to eat until satisfied.

In our laboratory at the University of Sydney, Dr. Susanna Holt developed the world's first **satiety** index of foods. Volunteers were given a range of individual foods that contained equal numbers of calories, and their satiety responses and their subsequent food intake were then compared.

Dr. Holt found that the most filling foods were those that contained fewer calories per gram—that is, those that had the least energy density. These included potatoes, oatmeal, apples, oranges, and pasta. Eating more of these foods satisfies appetite without providing excess calories. Foods that provided a lot of calories per gram, like croissants, chocolate, and peanuts, were the least satisfying. These foods are more likely to leave you wanting more and to lead to what scientists call passive overconsumption—overeating without realizing it.

A GI Success Story

"I TURNED SIXTY last year. When I saw the photos of myself at my surprise birthday party, I was shocked and dismayed at how heavy I'd become! So I began dieting and going to the gym five times a week. Well, that didn't work—I couldn't lose a pound! Then I attended a seminar about the glycemic index and sugars in foods, and it just "clicked" that I was going down the wrong path for weight loss. I began following a low-GI regime, coupled with my regular exercise regime, and now, a year after my sixtieth birthday, I'm forty-four pounds thinner!"

—Margaret

After energy density, the second best predictor of satiety was a food's GI value—the lower the GI value, the more the food satisfied people's hunger. Indeed, there are now more than twenty studies that confirm that low-GI foods are able to suppress hunger longer than high-GI foods.

There are probably several mechanisms responsible for this.

▶ Low-GI foods remain in the small intestine longer, triggering receptors that tell the brain there's food still in the gut to be digested. Many of these receptors are present only in the lower gut. It doesn't take a genius to appreciate that a food that empties rapidly from the stomach and gets digested and absorbed in minutes won't satisfy for hours on end.

- High-GI foods may stimulate hunger, because the rapid rise and then fall in blood glucose levels appears to stimulate counterregulatory responses to reverse the decline.
- Stress **hormones** such as adrenaline and cortisol are released when glucose levels rebound after a high-GI food is consumed. Both hormones tend to stimulate appetite.
- Low-GI foods may be more satiating simply because they are often less energy dense than their high-GI counterparts. The naturally high fiber content of many low-GI foods increases their bulk without increasing their energy content.

■ How Low-GI Diets Help You Lose Fat ■

Even when the calorie intake is the same, people eating low-GI foods may lose more weight than those eating high-GI foods. There are now at least ten studies showing that individuals eating low-GI foods lose more body fat than those eating normal high-GI foods (see the summary of these studies, "Low-GI Foods and Weight: A Summary of the Scientific Evidence," on pages 335–336 in the references section). Sometimes the result is not statistically different, but the trend is always in the direction that favors the low-GI diet.

In one study conducted by David Ludwig, MD, PhD, and Cara Ebbling, PhD, at Boston Children's Hospital, adolescents were instructed to follow either a conventional high-fiber, low-fat diet or a low-GI diet containing a little more protein and less carbohydrate. The low-GI group's diet emphasized foods such as oatmeal, eggs, low-fat dairy, produce, and pasta. In contrast, the low-fat diet emphasized whole-grain, high-fiber cereal products, potatoes, and rice. Both diets contained the same number of calories and were followed for twelve months. At the end of the first six months, the people in the group eating low-GI foods had lost 6.6 pounds (3 kilograms) of body fat, while the low-fat group lost none. Furthermore, at the end of that year, the low-GI group had maintained their fat loss, while the other group had gained weight.

In the Human Nutrition Unit at the University of Sydney, we have made similar findings in a group of overweight young adults. To ensure dietary compliance, we gave them most of the food they needed for the entire twelve-week period. At the end, we found that weight and body fat loss were 80 percent greater in those following the low-GI regimen than in those following the conventional low-fat approach.

How did the low-GI diet work? The most significant finding was the different effects of the diets on the level of glucose in the blood. Low-GI foods resulted in lower levels of both glucose and insulin over the course of the day and night.

Are Potatoes Fattening?

DESPITE THEIR HIGH GI value, potatoes are highly filling during the first two hours after consumption. One explanation for this is their low calorie content—to consume 250 calories, you would need to eat seven medium-sized potatoes. It is possible, however, that in the period three to four hours after consumption, the high insulin response caused by potatoes may cause lower levels of glucose and free fatty acids in the blood. In turn, this may increase the levels of the stress hormones cortisol and noradrenaline and thereby stimulate appetite—a finding that has been shown in previous studies.

Low-GI cooking tip: If potatoes are your favorite food, don't cut them out—instead, eat them in moderation, cut your usual portion in half and add a lower-GI accompaniment like sweet corn, or cook them ahead of time—then cool and reheat before eating (which lowers the GI). Steam small new potatoes (with their skin for added nutrients), or bake a potato and add a tasty, low-GI topping—again, sweet corn, beans, or chickpeas. Boiled potatoes or a simple potato salad made with a vinaigrette dressing have a lower GI and are a much better choice for weight control than French fries or potato chips, which are far higher in fat and calories. See part 4 for more suggestions about eating potatoes the low-GI way.

There are even more good reasons to choose low-GI carbs for weight loss. When people first begin a diet, their metabolic rate drops in response to their reduced caloric intake. One study found, however, that the metabolic rate had dropped less after one week on a low-GI diet than on a conventional high-carbohydrate diet. So the engine revs are higher. The same study suggested that the low-GI diet helped to preserve lean body mass better (and remember, muscle burns lots of calories and keeps your metabolism revved), which could explain the higher metabolic rate.

New research also provides evidence that low-GI diets are able to bring about a reduction in the dangerous fat—around the abdomen—with minimal loss of muscle. In a French study, overweight men were given, in succession, a high- and low-GI weight-maintaining diet (in random order), equivalent in energy and macronutrient composition. After five weeks on each diet, their body-fat mass was measured using sophisticated X-ray methods. Those allocated to the low-GI diet had lost one pound of fat from the abdomen. There was no difference in subcutaneous fat (the fat under the skin). That evidence was backed up by a large observational study in Europe of people with type 1 diabetes. It found that those who had followed a low-GI diet not only had better blood glucose control values, but the men in the group also had smaller waist circumferences, a good index of abdominal fat, or **central obesity**.

Large-scale studies in people with diabetes have found that diets including low-GI carbs are linked not only to smaller waist circumference but also to better diabetes control.

In the table below, foods of high and low energy density but equal caloric value are compared. On the left are small amounts of energy-dense foods that provide the same number of calories as the larger amounts of low-energy-dense foods on the right.

High-Energy-Dense Foods	Low-Energy-Dense Foods
2 Chips Ahoy chunky chocolate-chip cookies	2 graham crackers spread with light ricotta cheese and jam
A hot fudge sundae	A frozen fruit bar
An 8-ounce container of full-fat yogurt	An 8-ounce container of light yogurt and 1 banana
A snack pack of raisins	A small bunch (½ cup) of grapes and a medium-sized apple
6 Ritz crackers and cheddar cheese	2 Wasa crackers topped with ham, tomato, and cucumber
Small, medium, or large fries	1 large baked potato with ½ cup steamed broccoli, grated cheese, a small orange juice, and an apple

Weight Gain in Pregnancy

DID YOU GAIN a lot of weight during pregnancy and not lose it all afterward? A high-GI diet may be partially to blame. One study suggests that weight gain during pregnancy is influenced greatly by the GI values of the diet. Women who followed a low-GI diet from early on in pregnancy gained only twenty pounds, compared to forty-four pounds gained by those eating an otherwise equivalent high-GI diet. What's more, the baby's birth weight and body-fat content were also higher if the mother's diet was high GI. A recent Australian study published in the *American Journal of Clinical Nutrition* found a much higher rate of large-birth-weight babies (over ten pounds) in women consuming a higher-GI diet during pregnancy. It's been known for a long time that a baby's birth weight is related to the mother's blood glucose levels. Women with diabetes (or at risk of developing it) have heavier babies than those without diabetes. Now it seems that *all* the maternal tissues may respond to the high levels of glucose and insulin that occur after eating high-GI foods. That includes the fat stores laid down to sustain lactation. While we await more studies, low-GI diets during pregnancy can do no harm.

■ Four Key Tips for Losing Weight ■

1. Focus on what to eat, rather than what not to eat.

Typically, people approach weight management by looking at which foods they're supposed to eat less of. A better option is to focus on meeting your ideal fruit and vegetable intake first, and then see how much room you have left to fit in the extras.

Every day you need to eat at least the minimum of these foods:

Vegetables and legumes—at least 5 servings every day.
- 1 serving means:
  ½ cup cooked vegetables
  1 cup raw or salad vegetables
  1 small potato
  ½ cup cooked lentils, chickpeas, or beans

Fruit—at least 2 servings every day.
- 1 serving means:
  1 medium piece of fruit (apple, banana, or orange)
     or 2 small pieces of fruit (apricot, plum, kiwi)
  1 cup small fruit pieces
  ½ cup fruit juice
  ¼ cup dried fruit

Breads/cereals/rice/pasta and noodles—
4 servings or more every day.
- 1 serving means:
  1 ounce ready-to-eat cereal
  ½ cup cooked pasta, noodles, or rice
  ½ cup cooked cereal
  1 slice bread
  ½ bread roll

2. Eat at least one low-GI food at each meal.

Simply substituting low-GI foods for high-GI alternatives ("this for that," as we call it) will give your overall diet a lower GI and will reduce insulin levels and increase your body's fat-burning potential. Simply by replacing at least one high-GI carbohydrate choice at each meal with a low-GI type you can achieve an effective reduction in your insulin levels. It's the carbohydrate foods you eat the most of that have the greatest impact—so check the following table and put slow carbs to work in your day by cutting back consumption of high-GI foods and replacing them with low-GI alternatives that are just as tasty.

This for That

If you are currently eating this (high-GI) food	Choose this (low-GI) alternative instead
Cookies	A slice of whole-grain bread or toast with jam, fruit spread, or Nutella.
Breads such as soft white or whole wheat; smooth-textured breads, rolls, or scones	Dense breads with whole grains, whole-grain and stone-ground flour, and sourdough; look for low-GI labeling.
Breakfast cereals—most commercial, processed cereals including corn flakes, Rice Crispies, cereal "biscuits" such as shredded wheat	Traditional rolled oats, muesli, and the commercial low-GI brands listed on page 297; look for low-GI labeling.
Cakes and pastries	Raisin toast, fruit loaf, and fruit buns are healthier baked options; yogurts and low-fat mousses also make great snacks or desserts.
Chips and other packaged snacks such as Twinkies, pretzels, Pop-Tarts	Fresh grapes or cherries, or dried fruit and nuts.
Crackers	Crisp vegetable strips such as carrot, pepper, or celery.
Doughnuts and croissants	Try a skim milk cappuccino or smoothie instead.
French fries	Leave them out! Have salad or extra vegetables instead. Corn on the cob or coleslaw are better fast-food options.
Candy	Chocolate is lower GI but high in fat. Healthier options are raisins, dried apricots, and other dried fruits.
Muesli bars	Try a nut bar or dried fruit and nut mix.

If you are currently eating this (high-GI) food	Choose this (low-GI) alternative instead
Potatoes	Prepare smaller amounts of potato and add some sweet potato or sweet corn. Canned new potatoes are an easy and lower-GI option. You can also try sweet potato, yam, taro, or baby new potatoes—or just replace with other low-GI or no-GI vegetables.
Rice, especially large servings of it in dishes such as risotto, rice salads, fried rice	Try basmati or Uncle Ben's converted long-grain rice, Japanese sushi rice with salmon and vinegar, barley, cracked wheat (bulgur), quinoa, pasta, or noodles.
Soft drinks and fruit juice drinks	Use a diet variety if you drink these often. Fruit juice has a lower GI (but it is not a lower-calorie option). Water is best.
Sugar	Moderate the quantity. Consider pure floral honey (not commercial blends), apple juice, fructose, and grape nectar as alternatives.

3. Reduce your fat intake, especially saturated fat.

Because fat contains more calories per gram than any other food (in other words, it's more energy dense), it can provide lots of calories without making you feel full. It is, however, unnecessary and unwise to cut out fat completely. Instead, aim to reduce sources of saturated fat (butter, cream, cheese, cookies, cakes, fast foods, chips, sausages, most cold cuts, fatty meats) while maintaining a moderate consumption of foods high in unsaturated, healthier fats (most oils, margarines, nuts, avocados).

Remember, too, that while a low-fat diet is important, the calories from other sources are just as important. Rice and bread contain little fat, but when your body is burning the carbohydrate in these foods, it doesn't burn as much fat. So even if you do truly follow a low-fat diet, you won't lose weight if your caloric intake is still high.

High-GI Diets and Nonalcoholic Fatty Liver (NAFL) Disease

AS THE INCIDENCE of obesity in adults and children increases, so does nonalcoholic steatohepatitis (NASH) and **nonalcoholic fatty liver (NAFL) disease**. Both are caused by excess fat deposits in the liver and lead to inflammation or scarring. NASH and NAFL are strongly associated with insulin resistance and are relatively common in people with type 2 diabetes. Currently, the only effective treatment is weight loss, which makes timely the findings of a recent Italian study published in the *American Journal of Clinical Nutrition*.

In this study, the research suggests that a low-GI diet may help people with NAFL more than low-carb or high-fiber diets and can be a complementary tool for preventing or treating it. In their cross-sectional study of 247 healthy individuals, the researchers looked at dietary correlations with NAFL, assessing the effects of both the quality and quantity of carbohydrate. They found that the GI of the diet is a good marker for fatty liver. The higher the GI, the greater the prevalence of fatty liver, especially in insulin–resistant people. In an editorial in the same issue, Dr. David Jenkins, who first developed the GI, called for further studies to "assess whether a low-GI diet, given as an intervention, makes a difference in the natural history of NAFL."

Is Your Diet Too High in Fat?

USE THIS FAT counter to tally up how much fat your diet contains.

Circle all the foods that you could eat in a day, look at the serving size listed, and multiply the grams of fat up or down to match your serving size. For example, with milk, if you estimate you might consume 2 cups of regular milk in a day, this supplies you with 20 grams of fat.

Food	Fat content (grams)	How much did you eat?
DAIRY FOODS		
Milk, 1 cup		
whole	8	_____
2%	5	_____
1%	3	_____
fat free (skim)	0	_____
Yogurt, 8-ounce container		
regular	7	_____
nonfat	0	_____
light or low fat	2–3	_____
Ice cream, vanilla, ½ cup		_____
regular	7	_____
reduced fat	2	_____
Cheese		
American, regular, 1 oz	9	_____
American, low fat	3	_____
Cottage cheese, 2%, 2 tablespoons	1	_____
Ricotta, 2 tablespoons		
whole milk	8	_____
part skim	3	_____
light	2	_____
Cream/sour cream, 1 tablespoon		
regular	2	_____
reduced fat	1	_____
fat free	0	_____
FATS AND OILS		
Butter/margarine, 1 teaspoon	4	_____
Oil, any type, 1 tablespoon	14	_____

Food	Fat content (grams)	How much did you eat?
Cooking spray, ⅓-second spray	0	_____
Mayonnaise, 1 tablespoon		
regular	11	_____
light	5	_____
cholesterol free	5	_____
Salad dressing, 2 tablespoons		
regular	5–10	_____
reduced fat	2–5	_____
MEAT		
Beef, 5 ounces		
top sirloin	12	_____
ground, lean	18	_____
top round roast	9	_____
London broil	9	_____
Pork		
baked ham, 5 oz	8	_____
sausage, 2 oz	8	_____
tenderloin, 5 oz	9	_____
center cut, 5 oz	12	_____
bacon, 3 strips	9	_____
Veal		
cutlets, 5 oz	9	_____
Lamb		
leg, roast, 5 oz	12	_____
Chicken		
breast, skinless, 5 oz	6	_____
drumstick, with skin, 2 oz	6	_____
thigh, with skin, 2½ oz	10	_____
nuggets, breaded & fried, 6 pieces	20	_____
FISH		
Grilled fillet, 3 oz	1	_____
Salmon, 3 oz	11	_____
Fish sticks, breaded & fried, 3 oz	10	_____

Food	Fat content (grams)	How much did you eat?
SNACK FOODS		
Chocolate bar, 1 oz	5	_____
Potato chips, 1 oz	10	_____
Tortilla chips, 1 oz	10	_____
Peanuts, 1 oz	14	_____
French fries, 10 pieces	4	_____
Pizza, cheese, 1 slice, 4 oz	11	_____
Pretzels, 1 oz	1	_____
TOTAL		_____

HOW DID YOU RATE?

< 40 grams Excellent. Thirty to 40 grams of fat per day is an average range recommended for those trying to lose weight.

41–60 grams Good. A fat intake in this range is recommended for most adult men and women.

61–80 grams Acceptable if you are very active, i.e., doing hard physical work or athletic training. It is too much if you are trying to lose weight.

> 80 grams You're possibly eating too much fat, unless of course you are Superman or Superwoman!

4. Eat regularly.

Recent evidence strongly indicates that people who graze properly—eating small amounts of nutritious food throughout the day at frequent intervals—may actually be doing themselves a favor. Specifically, researchers compared people who ate three meals a day versus those who ate three meals and three snacks. They showed that snacking stimulated the body to use up more energy for metabolism than concentrating the same amount of food into three meals. It's as if the more often you give your body fuel, the more it will burn.

The problem with grazing is that often we turn to high-fat foods like cakes, chocolate, candy bars, chips, or pastries, all of which add empty calories and little or no nutritional value. Another criticism is that for those who tend to overeat, increasing the number of times they face food is courting disaster. Choosing low-GI snacks will reduce your chance of overeating. Using our snack suggestions (see "Snacks—Making the Right Between-Meal Choices" on page 206), you can enrich the variety of foods in your diet and feel satisfied before you have eaten too much. Measure out your portions and eat slowly.

Every day you also need to accumulate sixty minutes of physical activity (including incidental activity and planned exercise).

■

The evidence from people who have lost weight and maintained their weight loss over the long term is that there is no magic bullet. Rather, they:

- **wanted to change their diet to improve their health**
- **were willing to lose weight slowly**
- **made lasting changes to their diet and activity patterns**

■

In part 4, Your Guide to Low-GI Eating, we show you how to make the change to a low-GI diet along with the low-GI food finder, pantry planner, cooking tips, and more than 45 delicious recipes making the most of low-GI ingredients.

For our twelve-week, low-GI weight-loss program, we encourage you to consult *The Low GI Diet Revolution* and *The Low GI Diet Cookbook: 100 Simple, Delicious Smart-Carb Recipes—The Proven Way to Lose Weight and Eat for Lifelong Health.*

Make Healthy Eating a Habit

MAKE HEALTHY EATING a habit. Motivation is what gets you started. Habit is what helps to keep you going. Some key tips:

- Make breakfast a priority.
- If it's healthy keep it handy.
- Don't buy food you want to avoid.
- Make sure temptation is more than an arm's length away—"plate" dishes in the kitchen (as a restaurant would) before sitting down at the table.
- Listen to your appetite—eat when you are hungry and stop when you are full (you don't have to leave a clean plate).

· 7 ·

The Glycemic Index
and Diabetes

*D*iabetes is on its way to becoming one of the most serious and most common health problems in the world. A diabetes epidemic is gaining momentum in many developed and newly industrialized nations; worldwide, over the last twenty years, the total number of people with diabetes has risen from 30 million to 230 million, and the International Diabetes Federation predicts it will affect 350 million people by 2025.

In some developing countries, half of the adult population already has diabetes. Even in developed countries, the rate of diabetes is increasing at an alarming rate. Nearly 21 million Americans have diabetes—with more than 6 million of them unaware that they have the disease. Forty-one million Americans are estimated to have prediabetes, the precursor condition to diabetes, and at current rates of growth, more than 10 percent of all Americans will have diabetes by 2010. In the absence of any sort of preventive intervention, everyone with prediabetes will eventually develop diabetes.

The glycemic index has far-reaching implications for diabetes and prediabetes. Not only is it important in treating people with diabetes, but it may also help prevent people from developing diabetes in the first place, and possibly even prevent some of the **complications** of diabetes.

■ What Is Diabetes? ■

Diabetes is a chronic condition in which there is too much glucose in the blood. Keeping the glucose level normal in the blood requires the right amount of a hormone called **insulin**. Insulin gets the glucose out of the blood and into the body's muscles, where it is used to provide energy for the body. If there is not enough insulin, or if the insulin does not do its job properly, diabetes develops.

Type 1 diabetes (formerly referred to as insulin-dependent diabetes, or juvenile diabetes) is an **autoimmune disease** triggered by as yet unknown environmental factors (possibly a virus) that usually develops in childhood or early adulthood. In type 1 the **pancreas** cannot produce enough insulin, because the body's **immune system** has attacked and destroyed its insulin-producing **beta cells**. Five to 10 percent of people with diabetes have type 1 diabetes (about 1 million people in the United States). To survive, people with type 1 require insulin, delivered through injections or an insulin pump.

Type 2 diabetes (formerly known as non-insulin-dependent diabetes) is largely inherited, but overeating, being overweight, and not exercising enough are important lifestyle factors that can lead to this type of diabetes, particularly in those with a family history of diabetes. Ninety to 95 percent of people with diabetes have type 2.

Typically, type 2 diabetes develops after the age of forty. But our society's increasing physical inactivity and obesity has led to diagnoses in younger and younger people; particularly in some ethnic groups, even children less than ten years of age are developing type 2.

People develop type 2 diabetes because they have developed **insulin resistance**, which means that their body is less sensitive, or "partially deaf," to insulin. The organs and tissues that ought to respond to even a small increase in insulin remain unresponsive. So the body tries harder by secreting more insulin to achieve the same effect. This is why high insulin levels are central to insulin resistance. (For more about insulin resistance, see "Understanding the Metabolic Syndrome and Insulin Resistance," pages 117–118.

Initially in people with type 2, the body struggles to make extra insulin; left untreated, they develop a shortage of insulin. Treatments for type 2 aim for people to make the best use of the insulin their bodies produce and to try to make it last as long as possible. In some cases, oral medications or exogenous insulin (from injections or, as of late 2006, inhaled) may be necessary to treat this type of diabetes.

■ Prediabetes, the Precursor Condition for ■ Diabetes and a *Risk Factor* for Heart Disease

An estimated 40 million Americans have **prediabetes**, which is about twice the number of people in the United States who have diabetes. People with prediabetes (formerly described as having "a touch of diabetes," "a touch of sugar," or "**impaired glucose tolerance**") occupy a kind of middle ground between people with normal **fasting blood glucose levels** and those with diabetes:

Normal Fasting Blood Glucose: < 100 mg/dL
   (< 5.6 mmol/L)
Prediabetes Fasting Blood Glucose: 100–125 mg/dL
   (5.6–6.9 mmol/L)
Diabetes Fasting Blood Glucose: > 125 mg/dL (> 6.9 mmol/L)

Prediabetes is a major public health issue; many people with the condition (up to 50 percent) will develop diabetes if they do not make lifestyle changes that will help control their blood glucose levels: improving diet, increasing activity levels, and losing weight. Having prediabetes also increases the risk of heart disease and stroke.

■ How to Know If You Are at Risk ■ of Prediabetes or Type 2 Diabetes

If any of the following statements apply to you, then your blood glucose should be checked regularly, as blood glucose testing is the only way of finding out if you have prediabetes or diabetes. Arrange the appropriate tests through your doctor.

▶ You're over the age of fifty-five.
▶ You have a family history of diabetes.
▶ You're overweight.
▶ You have high blood pressure.
▶ You've had diabetes during pregnancy (gestational diabetes).
▶ You're from one of the following ethnic backgrounds: Native American, Puerto Rican, Mexican American, African American, Cuban, or Pacific Islander.

If you don't know if one or more of these statements applies to you, make an appointment with your doctor for a checkup.

If one or more of these does apply to you, you can reduce your chances of developing diabetes by controlling your weight, exercising more, and eating more foods with low GI values. Reducing the GI value of the foods you eat reduces the demand on your pancreas to produce more insulin, perhaps prolonging its function and delaying the development of diabetes. Research done by Harvard University has shown that eating low-GI foods that are high in fiber is associated with the lowest risk of developing type 2 diabetes. Another study, by Swedish researchers, found that a diet rich in low-GI foods and fiber improved insulin levels in people at risk for developing diabetes.

■ What Is Insulin Resistance? ■

Insulin resistance means that your body is insensitive, or "partially deaf," to insulin. The organs and tissues that ought to respond to even a small increase in insulin remain unresponsive. So your body tries harder by secreting more insulin to achieve the same effect. This is why high insulin levels are part and parcel of insulin resistance. You probably have insulin resistance if you have two or more of the following:

▶ high blood pressure
▶ low HDL-cholesterol levels

- large waist circumference
- high uric acid levels in blood
- prediabetes
- fasting glucose ≥ 110 mg/dL (6.1 mmol/L)
- postglucose load ≥ 140 mg/dL (7.8 mmol/L)
- high triglycerides

Chances are your total cholesterol levels are within the normal range, giving you and your doctor a false impression of your coronary health. You might also be at a normal weight but have a large waist circumference (> than 31.5 inches [80 cm] in women, > 37 inches [94 cm] in men), indicating excessive fat around the abdomen. But the red flag is that your blood glucose and insulin levels after a glucose load, or after eating, remain high. Resistance to the action of insulin is thought to underlie and unite all the features of this cluster of metabolic abnormalities.

Why is insulin resistance so common? Genes and environment each play a role. People of Asian and African American origin and the descendants of the original inhabitants of Australia and North and South America appear to be more insulin resistant than those of Caucasian extraction, even when they are still young and lean. But regardless of ethnic background, insulin resistance develops as we age—probably because as we grow older, we gain excessive fat, become less physically active, and lose some of our muscle mass.

Diets with too little carbohydrate and too much fat (especially saturated fat) can make us more insulin resistant. If carbohydrate intake is high, eating high-GI foods can worsen preexisting insulin resistance.

Insulin resistance gradually lays the foundations of a heart attack and other diseases—stroke, polycystic ovarian syndrome (PCOS), fatty liver, acne, and cognitive impairment.

■ What About Gestational Diabetes? ■

Gestational diabetes is the type of diabetes that some women develop during pregnancy. In gestational diabetes, the body does not adapt to the hormonal changes set in motion during pregnancy, insulin resistance develops, and if the mother's body cannot produce enough insulin, the blood glucose levels are elevated above normal levels.

After most women with gestational diabetes give birth, their blood glucose levels return to normal and the gestational diabetes disappears. However, the risk of developing permanent diabetes later in life is very high. Women who have had gestational diabetes need to be proactive about reducing their chance of developing diabetes and should be checked regularly for diabetes.

In the United States, about 5 percent, or one in every twenty pregnant women, develops gestational diabetes, and those numbers are increasing. Gestational diabetes is more common in women of Native American, Hispanic, African American, Asian American, or Pacific Islander descent, and in women who are over thirty and who have previously had gestational diabetes.

Undetected and untreated gestational diabetes places a woman's baby at risk of serious medical complications. One of the most widely recognized is the risk of becoming too fat during pregnancy, which can make delivery difficult. Babies of mothers with gestational diabetes are at increased risk of other complications and are more likely to be overweight as children and to develop other health problems (e.g., high blood pressure, heart disease, and diabetes) later in life.

■ Why Do People Develop Diabetes? ■

As our ancestors began to grow food crops ten thousand years ago, their diet was no longer protein-based but rather carbohydrate-based, in the form of whole cereal grains, vegetables, and beans. Such a dietary change would also have changed the glucose levels in their blood. While they ate a high-protein diet, the glucose levels in their blood would not have risen significantly after a meal.

When our ancestors started eating carbohydrate regularly, their blood glucose levels would have increased after meals. The amount by which the glucose levels in the blood increased after a meal would have depended on the GI value of the carbohydrate. Crops such as spelt wheat grain, which our ancestors grew, had a low GI value. These foods would have had a minimal effect on glucose levels in the blood and the demand for insulin would have been similarly low.

As we also discussed in chapter 3, the second major change in our diet came with industrialization and the advent of high-speed steel-roller mills in the nineteenth century. Instead of whole-grain products, the new milling procedures produced highly refined carbohydrate, which we now know increases the GI value of a food and transforms a low-GI food into one with a high GI value. When this highly refined food is eaten, it causes a greater increase in blood glucose levels. To keep blood glucose levels normal, the body has to make large amounts of insulin. The vast majority of the commercially packaged foods and drinks that most people eat today have a high GI value. All of this strains the body's insulin-making capabilities.

Our bodies adapt to such major changes in diet over long periods of time. Because our European ancestors had thousands of years to adapt to a diet with a lot of carbohydrate, they were in a better position to cope with the changes in the GI values of foods. We believe that's why people of European descent have a lower prevalence of type 2 diabetes than people whose diets have recently changed to include lots of high-GI foods. There is, however, only so much that our bodies can take. As we continue to consume increasing quantities of foods with high GI values, plus excessive amounts of fatty foods, our bodies are coping less well. The result can be seen in the significant increase of people developing diabetes.

Large-scale studies at Harvard University, in which thousands of men and women have been studied over many years (see page 116 for more information about these studies), have shown that people who ate large amounts of refined, high-GI foods were two to three times more likely to develop type 2 diabetes or heart disease. The most dramatic increases in diabetes, however, have occurred in populations that have been exposed to these lifestyle changes over a much shorter period of time. In some groups of Native Americans and populations within the Pacific region, up to one adult in two has diabetes because of the rapid dietary and lifestyle changes they have undergone in the twentieth and twenty-first centuries.

■ Treating Diabetes ■

Watching what you eat is essential if you have diabetes. For some people with type 2 diabetes, diet, along with exercise, is *the* most critical way to keep their blood glucose levels in the normal range (70–110 mg/dL; 3.9–6 mmol/L). Others also need to take medicine or insulin. Everyone with type 1 diabetes must receive insulin, no matter what their diet. Regardless of the type or degree of their diabetes and their doctor-approved treatment, everyone with diabetes must carefully consider what they eat in order to keep their blood glucose levels under control. Research incontrovertibly shows that good (also called "tight") blood glucose control helps to prevent the dire **complications** that can arise: heart attacks, strokes, blindness, kidney failure, and leg amputations.

It wasn't until the 1970s that carbohydrate was considered to be a valuable part of the diabetic diet. Researchers found that a higher carbohydrate intake brought both improved nutritional status and insulin sensitivity. In the early 1980s, with Dr. David Jenkins's development of the glycemic index, as we described in chapter 2, the foundations were established for our present-day understanding of the real effect of those carbohydrates on blood glucose levels.

Some people think that because carbohydrate raises blood glucose levels, it should not be eaten at all by people who have diabetes. We cannot stress enough that this is simply not correct. We hope this is extremely clear by now: carbohydrate is an essential component of a healthy diet and helps maintain insulin sensitivity and physical endurance. Mental performance is also better when meals contain carbohydrate rather than just protein and fat. (See "Carbohydrate Is Brain Food" on pages 42–43).

Fundamentally, the GI demonstrates that the way for people with diabetes to incorporate more carbohydrates into their diet—without increasing their blood glucose levels—is to choose low-GI carbs.

Lowering the GI of your diet is not as hard as it seems, because nearly every carbohydrate food that we typically consume has an equivalent food with a low GI value. Our research has shown that blood glucose levels in people with diabetes are greatly improved if foods with a low GI value are substituted for high-GI foods—the "This for That" approach we talked about in the previous chapter (see pages 80–81).

We studied a group of people with type 2 diabetes and taught them how to alter their diets by replacing the high-GI foods they normally ate with low-GI carbohydrate foods. After three months we found a significant drop in their average blood glucose levels. They did not find the diet at all difficult; rather, they commented on how easy it had been to make the change and how much more variety had been introduced into their diet.

The Optimum Diet for People with Diabetes

- A low-fat, low-GI diet emphasizes lots of whole-grain breads (made with intact kernels); cereals like oats, barley, couscous, cracked wheat; legumes like kidney beans and lentils; and all types of fruits and vegetables.
- Only small amounts of fat, especially saturated fat. Limit cookies, cakes, butter, potato chips, take-out fried foods, full-fat dairy products, fatty meats, and sausages, which are all high in saturated fat. The poly- and monounsaturated olive, canola, and peanut oils are healthier types of fats.
- A moderate amount of sugar and sugar-containing foods. It's okay to include your favorite sweetener or sweet food—small quantities of sugar, honey, maple syrup, jam—to make meals more palatable and pleasurable.
- Only a moderate quantity of alcohol. Only two drinks for men and one drink for women per day, with at least two alcohol-free days a week.
- Only a moderate amount of salt and salted foods. Try lemon juice, freshly ground black pepper, garlic, chili, herbs, and other flavors instead of relying on salt.

Similar results have been reported by other researchers studying both type 1 and type 2 diabetes. For example, large studies in Australia, Europe, and Canada of people with type 1 diabetes have shown that the lower the GI of the diet, the better the diabetes control. The improvement in diabetes control seen after changing to a low-GI diet is often better than that achieved with some of the newer, expensive diabetes medications and insulins. Making this type of change in your everyday diet does not mean that your diet has to be restrictive or unpalatable. The recipes in part 4 of this book will show you how to reduce the overall GI value of your diet.

Many people with type 2 diabetes end up taking oral medication and/or insulin to control blood glucose levels. An increased intake of low-GI carbs can sometimes make these drugs unnecessary. Sometimes, however, despite your best efforts with diet, medication will be necessary to obtain good blood glucose control. This is eventually the case for most people with type 2 diabetes as they grow older and their insulin-secreting capacity declines further.

For more ideas about eating the low-GI way in your management of diabetes or prediabetes, see part 4, Your Guide to Low-GI Eating.

You also may find it helpful to consult *The New Glucose Revolution Low GI Guide to Diabetes* or other books in our series that include many recipes, including *The New Glucose Revolution Life Plan* and *The New Glucose Revolution Low GI Vegetarian Cookbook*.

A GI Success Story

"I WAS DIAGNOSED with type 2 diabetes a little over a year ago. The diet that my local diabetes association recommended wasn't working, and my symptoms—including blurry vision, weight gain, and high blood pressure—weren't getting better. Then, six months ago, I came across *The New Glucose Revolution* and began following a low-GI diet. Since then, I gradually reduced my insulin requirements until I no longer needed them. Today, my blood pressure and weight are back to normal, and my liver, kidney, and urine tests yielded a healthy result. Following a GI diet approach has truly helped me manage my diabetes, and I plan on eating this way for the rest of my life."

—John

■ The Dreaded Diabetes Complications ■

As we mentioned above, heart attacks, leg amputations, strokes, blindness, and kidney failure are more common in people with diabetes. The reason: poor blood glucose control can cause damage to the blood vessels in the heart, legs, brain, eyes, and kidneys—all parts of the body that are susceptible to microvascular damage. Poor blood glucose control can also damage the nerves in the feet, leading to pain and irritation, numbness, and loss of sensation.

In addition to high blood glucose levels, many researchers believe that high levels of insulin also contribute to the damage of the blood vessels of the heart, legs, and brain. High insulin levels are thought to be one of the factors that might stimulate muscle in the wall of blood vessels to thicken. Thickening of this muscle wall causes the blood vessels to narrow and can slow the flow of blood to the point that a clot can form and stop blood flow altogether. This is what happens to cause a heart attack or stroke.

We know that high-GI foods cause the body to produce larger amounts of insulin, which results in higher levels of insulin in the blood. Eating low-GI foods not only helps to control blood glucose levels, but it also does so with lower levels of insulin. Lower levels of blood glucose and insulin may have the added benefit of reducing large-vessel damage, which accounts for many of the problems that people with diabetes tend to experience.

■ The GI and Snacks ■

The GI is especially important when carbohydrate is eaten by itself and not as part of a mixed meal. Carbohydrate tends to have a stronger effect on blood glucose level when it is eaten alone rather than as part of a meal with protein foods, for example. This is the case with between-meal snacks, which most people with diabetes eat.

Many people taking insulin or oral medications need to eat some form of carbohydrate between meals to prevent their blood glucose from dropping too low (although newer forms of medication have lessened the likelihood of your needing to do this). Snacks, when chosen wisely, can make a significant nutrient contribution even if you're not taking any diabetes medication. We recommend them especially for small children, to ensure a sufficient caloric intake. Even for adults, regular snacks can prevent extreme hunger and help to reduce the amount of food eaten at a single sitting, which can help blood glucose control.

Studies that have looked at the metabolic effects of small, frequent meals (rather like grazing) versus two or three large meals each day have found that in people with type 2 diabetes, blood glucose and blood fat levels improve when meal frequency increases. There's also evidence that you will reap metabolic benefits by eating at regular set times rather than haphazardly.

Snacking isn't a license to eat more food. Rather, it is a way to spread the same amount of food over more frequent and smaller meals. Research indicates that if you spread your nutrient load more evenly over the course of a day, you may reduce the need for insulin in the disposal and uptake of carbohydrates. Researchers have seen this effect in people without diabetes, too. Although it has not been proven by controlled trials, it may also be that small, frequent meals could reduce your risk of developing diabetes by reducing the periodic surges in insulin that follow large meals.

■ Choose Low-GI Foods ■
for a Between-Meal Snack

An apple, with a GI of 38, is better than a slice of white toast, with a GI of around 70, and will result in a smaller jump in the blood glucose level. Other low-fat, low-GI snack ideas include:

- a fruit smoothie
- a low-fat milkshake
- an apple
- low-fat fruit yogurt
- 5 or 6 dried apricot halves
- a small banana
- 1 or 2 oatmeal cookies
- an orange
- a scoop of low-fat ice cream in a cone
- a glass of low-fat milk

■ Hypoglycemia— ■
The Exception to the Low-GI Rule

We discuss hypoglycemia in greater detail in the next chapter, but we want to mention it here briefly because people with diabetes who use insulin or oral medication may sometimes experience **hypoglycemia**, which occurs when one's blood glucose levels drop below 70 mg/dL (3.9 mmol/dL), the lower end of the normal range. Symptoms of hypoglycemia differ among individuals but can include feeling hungry (even ravenous), shaky, sweating, rapid heart beat, and an inability to think clearly.

Hypoglycemia (also known as low blood sugar) is a potentially dangerous situation that must be treated immediately by eating 15 grams (½ ounce) of fast-acting carbohydrate food. To treat a "hypo," you should eat a high-GI food because you need to increase your blood glucose quickly—and high-GI carbs will digest quickly. If you're not ready or about to eat your next meal or snack, you should also have some low-GI carbohydrates, like an apple, to keep your blood glucose from falling again until you next eat.

To Treat a Hypo . . .

Raise your blood glucose levels quickly with rapid-acting carbohydrate:

- Glucose tablets or gels (10–20 grams)
- ½ cup regular (not diet) soda, fruit juice, or sweetened fruit beverage
- 4 large jelly beans or 7 small jelly beans
- 2–3 teaspoons of sugar

Follow within 15–20 minutes with carbohydrate foods that will maintain blood glucose levels:

- 1 slice of low-GI bread
- 1 banana or apple
- A container of unsweetened yogurt (6 or 8 ounces) or ½ a container of sweetened yogurt (3 or 4 ounces)
- 1 glass of low-fat milk

A GI Success Story

"I'M FIFTY-FOUR and the CEO of a very large public-sector organization, with all that that entails, including missed meals, incorrect eating (often a single meal at night), long work hours, stress, etc. After not feeling well for some time, I consulted my family doctor, who ordered blood tests. They showed a relatively mild onset of type 2 diabetes and a couple of other disorders that, in the scheme of things, were not what you would consider serious but all of which could be attributed to my crazy lifestyle.

My doctor referred me to a dietitian who, thankfully with my knowledge now, was well versed in the glycemic index.

Three months later I have lost almost 26 pounds, am within 5 pounds of my goal weight, and feel significantly improved health-wise in all respects—including my self-esteem. My wonderful wife has also lost about 15 pounds, and she, too, doesn't need to lose much more.

Although I have yet to go back for blood tests, neither I nor Penny, my dietitian, have any doubt that there will be a major improvement in the results, since I feel so much better. At my first appointment with Penny, I told her that I was not there just to lose some weight and reduce my type 2 symptoms. That was certainly the primary objective, but my main goal was to change for the long term my eating and lifestyle habits.

Thanks primarily to your book I now believe I have achieved that. Both the philosophy and the practice of the glycemic index are relatively simple and easy to understand and very much common sense."

—Paul

■ If You're Having Trouble Controlling ■ Your Blood Glucose Levels . . .

Many factors can affect your blood glucose levels—your total dietary intake, your weight, your stress levels, how much exercise you're getting, and the medications you're taking. So if you have diabetes and you're finding it hard to achieve "tight control" of your blood glucose, we cannot stress strongly enough how important it is to seek medical help. Many endocrinologists work with dietitian/nutritionists and certified diabetes educators; this diabetes care team can help you assess and better manage the balance of factors that, all together, determine how well you're controlling your diabetes.

A GI Success Story

LOW BLOOD SUGARS in the night were a particularly worrisome problem for Jane. Her evening insulin doses had been adjusted in an effort to stop her blood glucose from going too low at night, but she believed that experimenting with her supper carbohydrate could also help. After trying all sorts of different foods and many 3 AM blood tests, she found the answer that the glycemic index predicted would work— milk! Jane found that before going to bed, a large glass of milk rather than her usual plain crackers was easy to have and maintained her blood glucose at a good level through the night.

▪ 8 ▪

The Glycemic Index
and Hypoglycemia

*Y*our body needs to maintain a minimum threshold level of glucose in the blood at all times to keep the brain and central nervous system functioning. If for some reason blood glucose levels fall below this threshold (specifically, below 70 mg/dL [3.9 mmol/L], the low end of the normal range), you experience **hypoglycemia**. It derives from the Greek words "hypo" (meaning under) and "**glycemia**" (meaning blood glucose)—hence *blood glucose level below normal*.

If you already have diabetes and are treating it with medication, you probably already know all about hypoglycemia. If you don't have diabetes but you have vague health problems, including fatigue and depression, and you think you may have hypoglycemia or someone tells you that you probably have "low blood sugar," you need to see your doctor and get a proper diagnosis.

When blood glucose levels rise too quickly after eating, they cause an excessive amount of insulin to be released. This draws too much glucose out of the blood and causes the blood glucose level to fall below normal. The result is hypoglycemia.

Hypoglycemia causes a variety of unpleasant consequences, which can be severe; they include trembling, sweating, palpitations, dizziness, nausea, incoherent rambling speech, and lack of coordination. If rapidly digested carbohydrates are not immediately consumed, coma and even death may ensue.

◼

- ▶ **Hypoglycemia is far less common than once was thought in people who do not have diabetes.**
- ▶ **Hypoglycemia due to a serious medical problem is rare.**
- ▶ **The most common form is reactive hypoglycemia, which occurs after eating.**

◼

However, the diagnosis of true **reactive hypoglycemia** *cannot* be made simply on the basis of these symptoms. Instead, it requires the detection of low blood glucose levels when the symptoms are actually being experienced. A blood test is required to do this. (The doctor will take a blood sample from your arm and send it to a laboratory for analysis.)

Home blood glucose meters are not sufficient for the diagnosis of hypoglycemia in people without diabetes. Because it may be difficult—or almost impossible—for someone to be in the right place at the right time to have a blood sample taken while experiencing the symptoms, a **glucose tolerance (GTT)** test is sometimes used to try to make the diagnosis. This involves drinking pure glucose, which causes the blood glucose levels to rise. If too much insulin is produced in response, a person with reactive hypoglycemia will experience an excessive fall in their blood glucose level. Sounds simple enough, but there are pitfalls.

Testing must be done under strictly controlled conditions; low blood glucose is best demonstrated by measuring properly collected capillary (not venous) blood samples. If your doctor uses an oral glucose tolerance test to diagnose hypoglycemia, you have to continue it for at least three to four hours (the normal time is two hours). Your insulin levels would be measured at the same time.

■ Treating Hypoglycemia ■

The aim of treating reactive hypoglycemia is to prevent sudden large increases in blood glucose levels. If the blood glucose level can be prevented from rising quickly, then excessive, unnecessary amounts of insulin will not be produced and the blood glucose levels will not plunge to abnormally low levels.

Smooth, steady blood glucose levels can readily be achieved by switching from high-GI foods to low-GI foods. This is particularly important when you eat foods that contain carbohydrates by themselves. Low-GI foods like whole-grain bread, low-fat yogurt, and low-GI fruits are best for snacks.

A GI Success Story

"MY LIFE HAS always been controlled by my hypoglycemia attacks, which almost always occurred in the late afternoon. They were so bad that I couldn't go anywhere without a blood sugar 'fix' in my pocket, be it an apple, a packet of chocolate-covered nuts and raisins, or a carton of juice. The attacks were awful—I'd lose the ability to concentrate and often even to function because I was so shaky and fatigued—yet my doctors claimed nothing was wrong with me. Finally, I started following a diet that incorporated low-GI snacks or meals every two hours. Somewhat to my surprise, my hypoglycemia drastically improved. I still experience minor fluctuations in blood sugar from time to time, but I'll have a little yogurt or an apricot and feel better within minutes. A low-GI eating approach has truly changed my life."

—Anne

If you can stop the big swings in blood glucose levels, then you will not get the symptoms of reactive hypoglycemia, and chances are you will feel a lot better.

Notably, hypoglycemia due to a serious medical problem is rare. Such conditions require in-depth investigation and treatment of the underlying medical problem causing hypoglycemia. But having an irregular eating pattern is the most common dietary habit seen in people who have hypoglycemia.

To prevent reactive hypoglycemia, remember:

▸ Eat regular meals and snacks—plan to eat every three hours.
▸ Include low-GI carbohydrate foods at every meal and for snacks.
▸ Mix high-GI foods with low-GI foods in your meals—the combination will give an overall intermediate or medium GI.
▸ Avoid eating high-GI foods on their own for snacks—this can trigger reactive hypoglycemia.

▪9▪

The Glycemic Index,
Heart Health, and
Metabolic Syndrome

*H*eart disease is the single biggest killer of people in North America. According to the American Heart Association, every twenty-nine seconds an American has a heart attack or goes into cardiac arrest.

Most heart disease is caused by **atherosclerosis**, also referred to as "hardening of the arteries." Most people develop atherosclerosis gradually during their lifetime. If it occurs slowly it may not cause any problems at all, even into old age. But if its development is accelerated by one or more of many processes (such as high cholesterol or high blood glucose levels), the condition may appear much earlier in life and can cause heart attacks and other serious health crisis.

▪

Knowing your blood glucose level is just as important as knowing your cholesterol level to be able to ensure optimum heart health.

▪

Risk Factors for Heart Disease

Risk Factors You cannot change:

- Being male
- Being older
- Having a family history of heart disease
- Being postmenopausal
- Your ethnic background

Risk factors you can do something about:

- smoking
- high blood pressure
- having diabetes or prediabetes
- having high blood cholesterol, high triglycerides, and low levels of the "good" (HDL) cholesterol
- having elevated CRP (C-reactive protein) levels (a marker of low-grade chronic inflammation somewhere in the body)
- being overweight or obese, or having extra fat around your abdomen
- being sedentary

SMOKING

Smokers have more than twice the risk of heart attack as nonsmokers and are much more likely to die if they suffer a heart attack. Smoking is also the most preventable risk factor for heart disease. Smokers tend to eat fewer fruits and vegetables compared with nonsmokers (and thus miss out on vital protective antioxidant plant compounds). Smokers also tend to eat more fat and more salt than nonsmokers. While these dietary differences may put the smoker at greater risk of heart disease, there is only one piece of advice for anyone who smokes: quit.

HIGH BLOOD PRESSURE

High **blood pressure** is the most common heart disease risk factor. High blood pressure (**hypertension**) is harmful because it demands that your heart work harder and it damages your arteries.

An artery is a muscular tube. Healthy arteries can change their size to control the flow of blood. High blood pressure causes changes in the walls of arteries, which makes atherosclerosis more likely to develop.

Blood clots can then form and the weakened blood vessels can easily develop a thrombosis (clot) or rupture and bleed.

Treatments for high blood pressure have become more effective over the last thirty years, but it is only now becoming clear which types of treatment for blood pressure are also effective at reducing heart disease risk.

DIABETES AND PREDIABETES

Diabetes and prediabetes cause inflammation and hardening of the arteries. High levels of glucose in the blood, even short-term spikes after a meal, can have many undesirable effects and are a predictor of future heart disease.

A high level of glucose in the blood means:

- The cells lining the arteries take up excessive amounts of glucose.
- Highly reactive charged particles called "free radicals" are formed, which gradually destroy the machinery inside the cell, eventually causing the cell's death.
- Glucose adheres to cholesterol in the blood, which promotes the formation of fatty plaque and prevents the body from breaking down cholesterol.
- Higher levels of insulin develop, which in turn raise blood pressure and blood fats, while suppressing "good" (HDL) cholesterol levels.

High insulin levels also increase the tendency for blood clots to form. This is why so much effort is put into helping people with diabetes achieve normal control of blood glucose levels. Even when cholesterol levels appear to be normal, other risk factors, such as triglycerides, can be highly abnormal.

But you don't need to have diabetes to be at risk—even moderately raised blood glucose levels before or after a meal have been associated with increased risk of heart disease in normal "healthy" people.

HIGH BLOOD CHOLESTEROL

Cholesterol is vital for healthy cells. It is so important, our bodies can make most of the cholesterol we need—about 1,000 mg per day. But in certain circumstances, we make more than necessary. This causes the level of cholesterol in our blood to build up, and that's when we have a problem. When the body accumulates too much cholesterol, it is deposited on the walls of the arteries, which become bloated and damaged and may become blocked.

Atherosclerosis leads to reduced blood flow through the affected arteries. In the heart, this can mean that the heart muscle gets insufficient oxygen to provide the power for pumping blood, and it changes in such a way that it causes pain (particularly, central chest pain, or angina pectoris). Elsewhere in the body, atherosclerosis has a similar blood-flow-reducing effect: in the legs it can cause muscle pains during exercise; in the brain it can cause a variety of problems, from irregular gait to strokes.

An even more serious consequence of atherosclerosis occurs when a blood clot forms over the surface of a patch of atherosclerosis on an artery. This process of thrombosis can result in a complete blockage of the artery, with consequences ranging from sudden death to a small heart attack from which the patient recovers quickly.

The process of thrombosis can occur elsewhere in the arterial system, with outcomes determined by the extent of the thrombosis. The probability of developing thrombosis is determined by the tendency of the blood to clot versus the natural ability of the blood to break down clots (fibrinolysis). These two counteracting tendencies are influenced by a number of factors, including the level of glucose in the blood.

People who have gradually developed atherosclerosis of the arteries to the heart (which are called the coronary arteries) may gradually develop reduced heart function. For a while the heart may be able to compensate for the problem, so there are no symptoms, but eventually it begins to fail. Shortness of breath may occur, initially on exercise, and there may sometimes be swelling of the ankles.

Modern medicine has many effective drug treatments for heart failure, so this consequence of atherosclerosis does not now have quite the same serious implications it did in the past.

■ Why Do People Get Heart Disease? ■

Atherosclerotic heart disease develops early in life when the many factors that cause it have a strong influence. Over many decades doctors and scientists have identified the risk factors (what we call red flags) in healthy people as well as in those with established heart disease. Your risk of developing heart disease is determined by things you cannot change, such as genetic (inherited) factors, and things you can do something about.

Having high blood cholesterol is partly determined by our genes, which can "set" the cholesterol level slightly high and which we cannot change; and partly by lifestyle or dietary factors, which push it up further—which we can do something about.

A diet high in saturated fat is the biggest contributor. Diets recommended for lowering blood cholesterol are low in saturated fat, high in good carbohydrate (particularly whole grains), and high in fiber, including plant sterols—natural plant compounds that inhibit the absorption of cholesterol. Some vegetable oils are a rich source of these compounds, and new types of margarine may incorporate extra doses. While the quality of fat has been the traditional focus of dietary approaches, we are now learning that the quality of carbohydrate can play a vital role in reducing the risk of heart disease.

Body weight also affects your blood cholesterol. In most people, being overweight increases blood cholesterol, and losing weight can be helpful.

There are some relatively rare genetic conditions in which particularly high blood cholesterol levels occur. People who have inherited these conditions need a thorough examination by a specialist doctor followed by a rigorous cholesterol-lowering eating plan combined with drug treatment to reduce and control the risk of heart disease.

What about the good HDL cholesterol?

HDL (high-density lipoprotein) cholesterol seems to protect us against heart disease because it clears cholesterol from our arteries and helps its removal from our bodies. Having low levels of HDL in the blood is one of the most important markers of heart disease.

LDL cholesterol—the bad cholesterol

LDL (low-density lipoprotein) cholesterol does the most damage to the blood vessels—it's a red flag for heart disease.

What about triglycerides?

The blood also contains **triglycerides**, another type of fat linked to increased risk of heart disease. Having too much triglyceride is often linked with having too little HDL cholesterol. Although people can inherit having excess levels of triglycerides, it's most often associated with being overweight or obese.

CRP (C-reactive protein)

Scientists have recently established that CRP in the blood is a powerful risk factor for heart disease. A measure of chronic low-grade inflammation anywhere in the body, it is indicative of the damaging effect of high glucose levels and other factors on the blood vessel walls.

In women, CRP levels may predict future risk of heart disease more effectively than cholesterol levels. Considering CRP and cholesterol levels together is a superior way for doctors to sort out those at greater risk.

Studies at Harvard have shown that CRP levels are higher in women consuming high-GI/high-glycemic-load diets. That's one more good reason to choose low GI!

Being overweight or obese, or having extra fat around your abdomen

Overweight and obese people are more likely to have high blood pressure and diabetes. They are also at increased risk of developing heart disease. Some of that increased risk is due to high blood pressure, and the tendency to diabetes, but there is a separate, "independent" effect of the obesity.

When increased fatness develops, it can be distributed evenly all over the body or it may occur centrally—in and around the abdomen. The latter is strongly associated with heart disease. In fact, you can have "middle-age spread"—a potbelly or a "muffin midriff"—and still be within a normal weight range. But that extra fat around the middle is playing havoc with your metabolism. Abdominal fat increases our risk of heart disease, high blood pressure, and diabetes. In contrast, fat on the lower part of the body, such as hips and thighs, doesn't carry the same health risk.

Being sedentary

Many of us exercise infrequently and lead sedentary lives, with long hours at our desks or behind the wheel of our cars. People who aren't active or don't exercise have higher rates of death and heart disease compared to people who perform even mild to moderate amounts of physical activity. Even gardening or going for a walk can lower your risk of heart disease.

A Healthy Waist

THE INTERNATIONAL DIABETES Federation has established new criteria for defining metabolic syndrome that reduce waist circumference thresholds to make it easier for doctors to identify people who have the condition. (A person with metabolic syndrome will have abdominal obesity plus at least two of the following other risk factors: high triglycerides, low HDL cholesterol, elevated blood pressure, and/or increased blood glucose.) The recommended limits of waist measurement are:

For people of European origin
- Men   37 inches (94 cm)
- Women   31.5 inches (80 cm)

For people from South Asia and China
- Men   35.5 inches (90 cm)
- Women   31.5 inches (80 cm)

For people from Japan
- Men   33.5 inches (85 cm)
- Women   35.5 inches (90 cm)

More information is available at www.idf.org/home/.

Regular physical activity can:

- help lower blood pressure
- cut heart attack and diabetes risk
- reduce insulin requirements if you have diabetes
- help you stop smoking
- control weight
- increase levels of "good" HDL cholesterol
- keep bones and joints strong
- reduce colon cancer risk
- improve mood
- ease depression
- increase stamina
- increase flexibility

Exercise and activity speed up your metabolic rate (increasing the amount of energy you use), which helps to balance your food intake and control your weight. Exercise and activity also make your muscles more sensitive to insulin (you'll need less to get the job done) and increase the amount of fat you burn.

A low-GI diet has the same effect. Low-GI foods reduce the amount of insulin you need, which makes fat easier to burn and harder to store. Since body fat is what you want to get rid of when you lose weight, exercise or activity in combination with a low-GI diet makes a lot of sense.

The effect of exercise doesn't end when you stop moving. People who exercise have higher metabolic rates, and their bodies burn more calories per minute even when they are asleep.

■ Treating Heart Disease ■ and Secondary Prevention

When heart disease is detected, two types of treatment are typically given. First, the effects of the disease are treated (for example, medical treatment with drugs and surgical treatment to bypass blocked arteries); and, second, the risk factors are treated in order to slow down further progression of the disease.

Treatment of risk factors after the disease has already developed is secondary prevention. In people who have not yet developed the disease, treatment of risk factors is primary prevention.

■ Preventing Heart Disease: ■ Primary Prevention

Thankfully, more and more people have their blood pressure tested and are checked for diabetes regularly. Increasingly, blood-fat tests are done to check people's risk factors for heart disease as well. If you haven't been checked recently, ask your doctor for these tests.

A good health professional will offer lifestyle advice that can reduce your risk of heart disease, including stopping smoking, regular exercise, and eating a healthy diet. But often, people find it difficult to fol-low this advice for long. This is especially true if heart disease isn't an immediate and life-threatening problem. But remember that it's bet-ter to take steps to be healthy today than to wait until heart disease has dramatically impaired your health.

■ The Glycemic Index and Heart Health ■

The GI is vitally important for coronary health and the prevention of heart disease.

First, it has benefits for weight control, helping to curb appetite and preventing overeating and excessive body weight.

Second, it helps reduce post-meal blood glucose levels in both nor-mal and diabetic individuals. This improves the elasticity of the walls of the arteries, making dilation easier and improving blood flow.

Third, blood fats and clotting factors can also be improved by low-GI diets. Specifically, population studies have shown that HDL levels are correlated with the GI values and glycemic load of the diet. Those of us who self-select the lowest-GI diets have the highest and best levels of HDL—the good cholesterol.

Furthermore, research studies in people with diabetes have shown that low-GI diets reduce triglycerides in the blood, a factor strongly linked to heart disease. Last, low-GI diets have been shown to improve insulin sensitivity in people at high risk of heart disease, thereby helping to reduce the increase in blood glucose and insulin levels after normal meals.

■

By working on several fronts at once, a low-GI diet has a distinct advantage over other types of diets or drugs that target only one risk factor at a time.

■

■ GI and Heart Disease: ■ The Weight of Evidence

One major study provides the strongest evidence in support of the role of GI in heart disease. Conducted by Harvard University and commonly referred to as the **Nurses' Health Study**, this ongoing, long-term study follows over 100,000 nurses, who every few years provide their personal health and diet information to researchers at Harvard School of Public Health.

Harvard's Nurses' Health Study found that those who ate more high-GI foods had nearly twice the risk of having a heart attack over a ten-year period of follow-up compared to those eating low GI-diets. This association was independent of dietary fiber and other known risk factors, such as age and body mass index. In other words, even if fiber intake was high, there was still an adverse effect of high-GI diets on risk. Importantly, neither sugar nor total carbohydrate intake showed any association with risk of heart attack. That means there was no evidence that lower carbohydrate or sugar intake was helpful.

Determining Your Body Mass Index

YOU CAN USE the BMI calculator at www.nhlbisupport.com/bmi/ or calculate it as follows:

1. Multiply your weight in pounds by 705.
2. Divide that answer by your height in inches.
3. Divide that answer by your height in inches.

To find your BMI in metric, divide your weight in kilograms by your height in meters squared.

One of the most important findings of the Nurses' Health Study was that the increased risk associated with high-GI diets was largely seen in those with a **body mass index (BMI)** over 23. There was no increased risk in those under 23. The great majority of adults, however, have a BMI greater than 23; indeed, a BMI of 23 to 25 is considered normal weight. The implication therefore is that the insulin resistance that comes with increasing weight is an integral part of the disease process.

If you are very lean and insulin sensitive, high-GI diets won't make you more prone to heart attack. This might explain why traditional-living Asian populations, such as the Chinese, who eat high-GI rice as a staple food, do not show increased risk of heart disease. Their low BMI and their high level of physical activity work together to keep them insulin sensitive and extremely carbohydrate tolerant.

■ Understanding the Metabolic Syndrome ■ and Insulin Resistance

Surveys show that one in two adults over the age of twenty-five has at least two features of what is seen to be a silent disease: the **metabolic syndrome**, or **insulin resistance syndrome**. This syndrome (formerly called **syndrome X**) is a collection of metabolic abnormalities that can quietly increase your risk of heart attack. The list of features is getting longer and longer, and the number of diseases linked to insulin resistance is growing.

People with metabolic syndrome are three times as likely to have a heart attack or stroke compared with people without the syndrome, and they have a fivefold greater risk of developing type 2 diabetes (if it's not already present).

The metabolic syndrome is a cluster of risk factors for a serious heart attack, recognized as a "cardiovascular time bomb." Different health and medical groups have different definitions (and those definitions may be changing), but most American physicians follow the definition of the National Cholesterol Education Program (NCEP), administered by the National Heart, Lung, and Blood Institute. According to the NCEP, a person with metabolic syndrome will have any three of the following:

- **triglycerides** ≥ 150 mg/dL (≥ 1.7 mmol/L)
- **HDL cholesterol** < 40 mg/dL (< 1.0 mmol/L) for men and < 50 mg/dL (< 1.3 mmol/L) for women
- **blood pressure** ≥ 130 / 85 mmHg. (either one of the numbers)
- **fasting plasma glucose** ≥ 110 mg/dL (≥ 6.1mmol/L)

▶ **waist circumference** < 40 inches (102 cm) in men or < 34.5 inches (88 cm) in women

The key to understanding metabolic syndrome is insulin resistance, which we discussed in chapter 9. Tests on patients with the metabolic syndrome show that insulin resistance is very common. If your doctor has told you that you have high blood pressure and prediabetes (formerly you might have been advised you have "a touch of sugar" or "impaired glucose tolerance"), then you probably have the insulin resistance syndrome.

■ How Can the GI Help? ■

Research shows that low-GI diets not only improve blood glucose in people with diabetes, but they also improve the sensitivity of the body to insulin.

In a recent study, patients with serious disease of the coronary arteries were given either low- or high-GI diets before surgery for coronary bypass grafts. They were given blood tests before their diets and just before surgery, and during surgery small pieces of fat tissue were removed for testing. The tests on the fat showed that the low-GI diets made the tissues of these "insulin insensitive" patients more sensitive—in fact, they were back in the same range as normal control patients after just a few weeks on the low-GI diet.

In another study, young women in their thirties were divided into those who did and those who did not have a family history of heart disease—and had not yet developed the condition. They had blood tests followed by low- or high-GI diets for four weeks, after which they had more blood tests. When they had surgery (for conditions unrelated to heart disease), pieces of fat were removed and tested for insulin sensitivity. The young women with a family history of heart disease were insensitive to insulin originally (those without the family history of heart disease were normal), but after four weeks on the low-GI diet, their insulin sensitivity was back within the normal range.

In both studies, the diets were designed to try to ensure that all the other variables (total energy, total carbohydrates) were not different, so that the change in insulin sensitivity was likely to have been due to the low-GI diet rather than any other factor.

■

Recent research reported in the *British Journal of Nutrition* found that eating just one extra low-GI item per meal can lower blood glucose levels and reduce the risk of metabolic syndrome.

■

Work on these exciting findings continues, but what is known so far strongly suggests that a low-GI diet not only improves body weight and blood glucose in people with diabetes, but it also improves the body's sensitivity to insulin. It will take many years of further research to show that this simple dietary change to a low-GI diet will definitely slow the progress of atherosclerotic heart disease. In the meantime, it is already clear that risk factors for heart disease are improved by a low-GI diet. Low-GI diets are consistent with the other required dietary changes needed for prevention of heart disease. For an even more in-depth discussion of the metabolic syndrome, heart health, and the GI, you may want to consult *The New Glucose Revolution Low GI Guide to the Metabolic Syndrome and Your Heart: The Only Authoritative Guide to Using the Glycemic Index for Better Heart Health.*

And as we've already stressed, you'll find much dietary guidance about how to adopt and eat the heart-healthy, low-GI way in part 4 of this book, Your Guide to Low-GI Eating.

• 10 •

The Glycemic Index and Polycystic Ovarian Syndrome (PCOS)

*P*olycystic ovarian syndrome, or **PCOS**, is more common than you might think. Elements of the disease are believed to affect a whopping one in four women in developed nations; the severe form affects one in twenty. It is a health condition linked with hormone imbalance and insulin resistance. The signs range from subtle symptoms, such as faint facial hair, to a "full house" of symptoms—lack of periods, heavy body-hair growth, obstinate body fat, and infertility. They can occur at any age, and can even be seen in girls as young as ten or women as old as seventy. (Contrary to popular belief, PCOS does not suddenly disappear at menopause.) Not only are the symptoms bothersome, but PCOS has also been tied to an increased link of heart disease and type 2 diabetes. You may also see it referred to as polycystic ovarian disease, Stein-Leventhal syndrome, or functional ovarian hyperandrogenism.

Only a doctor can diagnose PCOS. If you have any of the following symptoms, you should see your physician and ask her to refer you to an endocrinologist for proper diagnosis and treatment:

- delayed (or early) puberty
- irregular or no periods
- acne
- excess body or facial hair
- unexplained fatigue
- hypoglycemia (low blood glucose) after meals. The most common symptoms are light-headedness, sweating, sudden fatigue, and a "butterflies in the stomach" feeling
- excess weight around the waistline
- infertility
- mood swings
- hot flashes in young women
- sleep disorders such as sleep apnea or insomnia
- recurrent spontaneous miscarriages
- inappropriate lactation
- drop in blood pressure on standing up or with exercise
- rough, dark skin in the neck folds and armpits, a mark of severe insulin resistance from any cause

It is vital to diagnose and treat PCOS as early as possible to prevent it from developing to the "full house" syndrome. Diagnosis involves a blood test showing that key hormones are abnormally high or low; for example, testosterone that is too high, or high levels of *luteinizing hormone* (LH), while the level of *follicle-stimulating hormone* is normal. You may also undergo an ultrasound examination to see if you have enlarged ovaries with cysts. In thin women, ultrasound through the abdominal wall will reveal a clear picture of the ovaries, but overweight women may require an internal ultrasound. Both procedures are painless. Notably, symptoms, blood test results, and ultrasound findings should be interpreted by a medical practitioner with experience in PCOS. Keep in mind that some women do not show the "classic" signs at all, which is why consulting a doctor who knows the many facets of PCOS is so important.

■ The Insulin Resistance—PCOS Link ■

Insulin resistance is a condition in which the body "resists" the normal actions of the hormone insulin—meaning that the body's response to insulin is defective. To overcome this, the body secretes more insulin than normal. Most women with PCOS have severe insulin resistance, and as a result, high insulin levels. The problem is that insulin stimulates the growth and multiplication of cells in the ovary—in particular, those that make up the bulk of the ovary in which the eggs are embedded-causing them to become cystic. This flooding of insulin leads to a vicious cycle of hormonal imbalances that create the symptoms of PCOS.

The receptors for insulin in the ovaries are different from those in other tissues; when blood insulin levels are high, the ovary or ovaries do not turn down insulin receptor numbers or reduce their activity. As a result, the action of insulin continues unabated, and ovarian cells grow and multiply and increase their metabolic activity. The result is excessive production of both male sex hormone (testosterone) and female sex hormone (estrogen). High testosterone levels in women bring about "male" characteristics in women, such as weight gain and excessive hair on the face and in other areas. Excess insulin and sex hormones also stimulate one of the areas in the brain called the hypothalamus, making it more sensitive and causing it to secrete more luteinizing hormone. This stimulates the ovaries' hormone production even more, causing a vicious cycle. Breaking that cycle is the key to managing PCOS successfully.

■

Insulin resistance leads to a vicious cycle of hormonal imbalances that create the symptoms of PCOS.

■

Insulin resistance is more common in some people than others—for example, people of Asian descent have been found to be more resistant than Caucasians. Native American, Australian Aboriginals, and Pacific Islanders are more insulin resistant than most. Not surprisingly, PCOS also runs in families, and may have a genetic link. Environmental factors such as diet and a lack of physical exercise may also play a role. We also know that weight gain can trigger insulin resistance and PCOS, as can certain steroid medications. While being overweight or obese increases the degree of insulin resistance, you can be very lean and still have PCOS.

Effective medical management of PCOS

Although there's no "cure" as such for PCOS, keeping the symptoms under control is well within your grasp by making some diet and lifestyle changes that will encourage hormonal balance. When you see your doctor, you'll find that any medical management is usually tailored to your symptoms and to some extent your priorities—regular periods, a much wanted pregnancy, or simply a reduction in facial hair. It usually involves lifestyle changes along with insulin-sensitizing medication, such as metformin, to:

- improve your PCOS symptoms—regulating menstrual cycles, reducing acne and excess hair growth
- achieve and maintain a healthy weight
- control your blood glucose and insulin levels
- balance your hormone levels
- boost fertility
- give you more control and quality of life

The one thing women with PCOS say again and again is that they feel "out of control"—gaining weight, being unable to get pregnant, growing an excessive amount of body hair in areas where it shouldn't be, and so on. The good news is that by making some basic lifestyle changes—like eating the right kinds of foods and exercising more—you'll find yourself back in the driver's seat again. An additional benefit of making these changes is that you will reduce your risk of developing diabetes and heart disease.

■ The Four Steps That Will ■
Help You Take Charge

Modest changes that are easy to incorporate into your life will help your quality of life improve dramatically and lead to fewer symptoms of PCOS. You need to:

1. manage your weight
2. eat the healthy, low-GI way
3. move more
4. take care of yourself

Manage your weight

Managing your weight is essential if you have PCOS. That's because being overweight increases insulin resistance and worsens the symptoms of PCOS. You don't need to lose a lot of weight—or body fat—to improve your symptoms. Studies show that losing as little as 5 percent of body weight can help control blood glucose levels, improve menstrual function, reduce testosterone levels, reduce excess hair growth, and lessen acne. How much weight does this actually mean? Well, if you're 220 pounds, this means losing about eleven pounds of body fat can make a difference; if you're 154 pounds, losing just eight pounds would bring about a change.

As you probably know, the cornerstone of reaching and maintaining a healthy weight is a matter of balancing your calorie intake with the calorie output, or calories burned, from whatever physical activity you do. To lose weight and shed fat, you need to eat less and move more. But that doesn't mean starving yourself. It means choosing the right foods, which are low-GI foods—the ones the body burns rather than stores as fat, and that keep you feeling satisfied and full all day long. Women who change to a low-GI diet say they feel fuller and are less tempted to snack on not-so-healthy food—a big help when you're trying to shed pounds.

So what's the healthiest way to lose weight? First of all, aim to lose body *fat* rather than simply *weight*. Put the scales away and get out the tape measure, or even go by how your clothes fit. Remember, muscle weighs more than fat—so as you begin to exercise more, you may be shedding fat but adding muscle, meaning the scale might not reflect just how much you're changing. Second, don't think about going on a restrictive diet, as it will only make you feel deprived and lead to a binge. Instead, incorporate low-GI foods into a moderate diet. Third, be patient; it takes time to lose weight. And last, get moving. Regular physical activity every day will not only help you get fit and trim, but will also improve your heart and bone health, reduce your risk of diabetes, and help you manage stress.

Eat the healthy, low-GI way

The glycemic index plays a key role in helping you beat PCOS symptoms, because it focuses on carbohydrates—their quantity and quality, and their overall effect on your blood glucose. Controlling your blood glucose levels is the first step to increasing your insulin sensitivity. If you base your diet on eating balanced low-GI meals, you will make it easier for your body to burn fat and less likely for the fat to be stored in places where you don't want it.

Eating the healthy, low-GI way means changing your eating habits in a way that will last you a lifetime, and eating the right foods—foods that will fill you up, give you more energy, improve your health, *and*, best of all, help manage and even reduce your PCOS symptoms. It also means enjoying what you eat, while eating in a way that helps to control your insulin levels—specifically, with a low-GI diet, as detailed throughout this book.

Your healthy, low-GI eating plan should include the following foods every day:

- fresh vegetables and salads
- fresh fruit
- truly whole-grain breads (with lots of grainy bits and/or made with intact kernels) and cereals
- low-fat dairy products or nondairy alternatives like soy
- fish, lean meat, chicken, eggs, legumes, and soy products
- small amounts of healthy fats such as nuts, seeds, avocado, olives, olive oil, canola oil, or peanut oil

If you find it hard to get started, get help from a registered dietitian (see "How to Find a Dietitian," on page 48).

Move more

Activity and exercise are crucial if you want to manage PCOS, as they help you control your weight, manage your insulin, and make a real difference in your health and energy levels. Ideally, you should try to fit in activity on most days. Research shows that just thirty minutes of moderate intensity exercise each day can help improve your health, lowering your risk of heart disease and diabetes, among numerous other health problems. Busy schedule? Break the thirty minutes down into two sessions of fifteen minutes or even three sessions of ten minutes, and you'll still enjoy the same benefits. That said, if you're trying to lose weight, the more you can exercise, the better!

A balanced exercise program, including aerobic, resistance or "strength" training, and flexibility/stretching exercises will give you the best results. And don't forget to vary your activities—the body becomes efficient at anything it does repeatedly, so after a while, you won't see results unless you vary the type of activity or intensity.

Take care of yourself

Eating well and being active are the cornerstones of managing PCOS, but there are a few other things you can do to help yourself. Stress reduction is at the top of the list. Stress is a part of life for most of us and can't be avoided. The key is to be able to manage it effectively—which is absolutely crucial for women with PCOS, because too much stress can affect hormonal balance, increase blood glucose levels, and lead to overeating. You can get a handle on the stress in your life by starting a regular exercise program, taking time out for activities you enjoy, and finding someone to talk to about your feelings. If need be, talk to a counselor or therapist. Enough good-quality sleep is also important. A lack of sleep—that means less than eight hours for the average person—can reduce immunity, increase stress hormones, and worsen insulin resistance. If you've cut down on stress, started exercising regularly, and don't drink alcohol or caffeinated beverages before bed but still have difficulty sleeping, see your physician to find out if you may have a sleep disorder, or if medication and/or cognitive behavioral therapy may help.

For more information, check out *The New Glucose Revolution Guide to Living Well with PCOS.*

·11·

Children
and the Glycemic Index

*H*elping your children eat well is one of the most important things you can do for them. In an environment where food is overly abundant and physical activity limited, the potential for energy imbalance is great—and the consequences are enormous. About 30 percent of children and teenagers in the United States are overweight—a statistic that reflects a more than threefold increase in the percentage of overweight children and adolescents since the mid-1960s.

Overweight children are at risk for sleep apnea, high blood pressure, and elevated blood fats. Many will also have elevated levels of circulating insulin, which is an early warning sign for the potential development of type 2 diabetes—a condition, as we've previously noted, once seen only in adults but now increasingly being diagnosed in children. And overweight children face adulthood with the prospect of cardiovascular disease and reduced longevity. As if this weren't enough, overweight children are often stigmatized as lazy, unhealthy, and less intelligent than children of normal weight. Loss of self-esteem and subsequent social isolation can make their lives miserable.

■ How Can the Glycemic Index Help? ■

There's no simple solution for overweight and obese children. But managing overweight and obesity in children is about altering energy balance. Energy (calorie, or **kilojoule**) intake has to decrease, and energy expenditure (physical activity) has to increase. Today's American diet tends to be too high in fat and quickly digested carbohydrate foods that don't truly satisfy hunger. Many of our starchy staples, like potato, white bread, breakfast cereals, and crackers, have very high GI values. So, too, do children's favorites such as mashed potatoes, Rice Krispies, Gatorade, and jelly beans. Because of their high GI values, it is easy to overconsume calories by eating these foods. In contrast, low-GI foods like pasta, yogurt, most fruits, and oatmeal cookies have been proven to be more filling and can reduce overeating.

In a study that looked at twelve obese teenage boys in the United States, eating low-GI meals significantly reduced their subsequent food intake compared to high-GI meals. The boys ate special breakfast and lunch meals that had either a low, medium, or high GI value, and then their food intake was measured during the remainder of the day. Researchers found that the boys ate twice as much food in the afternoon after a high-GI breakfast and lunch as they did after a low-GI breakfast and lunch. This difference in food intake corresponded with alterations in hormonal and metabolic changes thought to be responsible for stimulating excessive appetite.

In addition, the boys had higher levels of the hormones insulin, noradrenaline, and cortisol after the high-GI meals. The trouble is that the increased insulin response to high-GI carbohydrates may promote fat storage and obesity, and higher cortisol levels may result in increased appetite. Differences in these hormones are one possible explanation for significantly greater fat loss in a group of children prescribed a diet based on low-GI foods compared to those on a conventional low-fat diet. With the low-GI diet, the children were instructed to eat until they were full, to snack when hungry, and to eat low-GI carbohydrate, protein, and fat at every meal and snack. Body mass index and body weight decreased significantly more (over the four-month study period) in those on a low-GI diet.

We Can't Stress This Enough: The Importance of Physical Activity

AN INCREASE IN physical activity is crucial for weight management for children. This includes reducing sedentary behaviors (such as television viewing, time on the computer, and video games) and increasing planned and incidental activity (such as having your children help with household tasks, play outside, and dress themselves).

It helps enormously if parents are involved in physical activity themselves. You'll serve as a role model for your kids. For this reason, it's a great idea to plan family activities such as walks, swimming, bike rides, and soccer or baseball games. Make it fun!

If children learn to combine regular physical activity with healthy low-GI eating, they will be in top condition throughout their lives.

■ Key Dietary Guidelines for Children ■

A healthy diet for children should:

- maintain good health and growth
- satisfy their appetite
- encourage good eating habits
- promote varied and interesting meals and snacks
- accommodate a child's usual routines and activities
- maintain a healthy body weight

Children need to eat a wide variety of nutritious foods to grow and develop to their full potential. As a parent or guardian you can follow these dietary guidelines for childhood and teen nutrition:

- Encourage and support breast-feeding.
- Make sure that your child eats a wide variety of nutritious foods, particularly calcium- and iron-rich foods.
- Steer clear of low-fat diets for young children. (For teenagers,

diets low in saturated fat, as recommended for adults, are appropriate.)

▶ Encourage your child to drink plenty of water.

▶ Check your child's growth regularly, and provide appropriate food and physical activity to ensure normal growth and development.

▶ Allow your child to eat only moderate amounts of sugar and foods containing added sugars.

▶ Choose low-salt foods for your child.

▶ Be sure that your child eats plenty of breads, cereals, vegetables (including legumes), and fruits.

▶ Include lean meats, fish, and dairy foods in their daily diet.

▶ Follow these guidelines yourself so that children can imitate you.

■ Incorporating Low-GI Foods ■ into Your Child's Diet

The GI of a diet can be lowered easily using our "This for That" approach, where at least half of high-GI carbohydrate choices are swapped for low-GI carbohydrate foods (see pages 80–81).

Keep the following characteristics of children's eating behavior in mind when attempting changes in their diet:

Children tend to dislike new foods. It's normal for children, especially young children, to refuse new foods. Repeated exposure to new foods in a positive environment—meaning you're not forcing the food on them, but encouraging them to try it—increases their acceptance. But you have to persevere—at least five to ten tastes of the food may be needed before a child accepts it and is willing to eat it.

Most children are natural grazers. They usually like to have frequent meals and snacks throughout the day. It's not a good idea to make children eat everything on the plate, as this can encourage overconsumption. It is preferable that they learn to stay in tune with their appetite and eat according to it.

Children have small stomachs with high nutrient requirements.
Their food intake may vary considerably from meal to meal, but
studies show it remains surprisingly constant from day to day. As
long as the foods offered to children are nutritious, their appetite
is the best indicator of how much they need to eat. Be clear on
what your role is as the caregiver in relation to feeding your children. The American nutritionist Ellyn Satter expresses it well:
"Parents are responsible for what is provided to eat. Children are
responsible for how much, and even whether, they eat."

■ The Best Carbohydrate Choices ■

The following foods have low GI values, are high in micronutrients,
and provide very little saturated fat; we note the recommended number of daily servings for children ages four to eleven:

Cereal grains (3–6 servings per day). Whole-grain breads, oatmeal and barley, oats, popcorn, rice, rye, wheat, and anything
made from them, such as bread, breakfast cereals, flour, noodles,
pasta, polenta, ravioli, and semolina.

Fruits (2–4 servings per day). Apples, apricots, bananas, cherries,
grapes, kiwi fruit, oranges, peaches, pears, plums, and raisins.
Serve them whole, in salads, or as juices and smoothies.

Vegetables and legumes (2–5 servings per day). Vegetables and
legumes provide valuable amounts of vitamins, minerals, and fiber.
As we've previously emphasized, because most vegetables are very
low in carbohydrate, you can eat most without thinking about their
GI value. All legumes—including baked beans, chickpeas, kidney
beans, lentils, and split peas—are low-GI sources of carbohydrate.

Milk and milk products (2–3 servings per day). Low-fat milk and
dairy foods such as pudding, ice cream, and yogurt are excellent
sources of carbohydrate and calcium. Children under age two
should be given full-fat milk; low-fat varieties are suitable for
older children.

As we've stressed, balanced meals usually consist of a variety of foods, and we know that eating a low-GI food with a high-GI food produces an intermediate-GI meal. As with adults, it isn't necessary to give children low-GI foods alone.

If You Want to Give Your Kids a Head Start, Give Them Oatmeal for Breakfast

IN RECENT YEARS, numerous studies have shown that eating breakfast can improve speed in short-term memory tests, alertness (which may help memory and learning), and can improve mood, induce calmness, and reduce feelings of stress. Breakfast also helps schoolchildren perform better in creativity tests. Breakfast helps to replenish blood glucose levels, which is important, since the brain itself has no reserves of glucose, its main energy source. Reporting in *Physiology & Behavior* in 2005, Tufts University psychologists confirmed the findings of previous studies—that when kids eat breakfast they do better on tests that require processing brainpower for complex visual display (such as puzzles) than when they skip breakfast. Taking it a step further this time, the Tufts team gave the kids different breakfasts on different occasions—oatmeal and milk one day and Cap'n Crunch with milk another, and then compared the test results. They found that the sixty elementary school students performed better on a raft of tests after eating stick-to-the-ribs oatmeal rather than firing up on Cap'n Crunch. Children ages nine to eleven showed improvements in their spatial memory (things like puzzles, drawing, and geography, as well as some technical skills used in math and science); the six- to eight-year-olds listened better and also scored higher on spatial memory. The researchers believe that their results show that what kids eat for breakfast really matters. They note: "Due to compositional differences in protein and fiber content, glycemic scores, and rate of digestion, oatmeal may provide a slower and more sustained energy source and consequently result in cognitive enhancement compared to low-fiber, high-glycemic, ready-to-eat cereal."

■ The Role of Sugar in Your Child's Diet ■

Most children naturally enjoy sweet foods. Sweetness is not a learned taste; our first food, breast milk, is sweet. Infants smile when offered sweet liquids and foods, and reject sour and bitter tastes.

As we have previously discussed in chapter 1, the GI demonstrates that sugar is not the dietary demon that it once was made out to be. You and your children can enjoy sugar and foods containing sugar in moderation as part of a balanced, low-GI diet. Research shows that diets containing moderate quantities of added sugars tend to be richest in micronutrients. As we explained in chapter 3, sugar itself has only a moderate GI value, and many foods containing sugar, such as yogurt and flavored milk, are excellent sources of low-GI nutrition.

What is a moderate intake of sugar in a child's diet?

A moderate intake of refined sugar in a child's diet is between 7 and 12 level teaspoons a day. This reflects average consumption in children and includes the sugar in foods such as soft drinks, breakfast cereals, candy, ice cream, cookies, and jams, as well as what is added—to breakfast cereal, for example. Adding sugar to a well-balanced, low-GI diet can make foods more palatable and acceptable to children without compromising their nutritional intake or the benefits of the low-GI foods.

Here's What a Moderate Quantity of Sugar in a Ten-Year-Old Child's Diet Looks Like

THIS CHILD'S MENU provides 12 teaspoons of refined sugars. It provides 1,500 calories of energy, with 23 percent of energy from fat and 57 percent of energy from carbohydrate.

BREAKFAST
¾ cup of Cocoa Puffs with 4 oz 1% milk
½ banana
4 oz fruit juice

SNACK

1 Quaker chewy low-fat granola bar

1 cup 1% milk

LUNCH

1 ham and cheese with lettuce and tomato sandwich
(made from low-GI bread)

6–8 baby carrots

1 small apple

1 cup water

SNACK

2 small chocolate-chip cookies

1 fruit smoothie (made with ½ cup 1% milk and ½ cup sliced fruit)

DINNER

1 cup of spaghetti with tomato sauce and 3 small meatballs

green salad, tossed with a little dressing if desired

½ cup steamed string beans

½ cup pudding and 2–3 strawberries

water to drink

SNACK

1½ cups air-popped popcorn

■ What About Artificially Sweetened Products? ■

Artificially sweetened products may be useful for some children in some circumstances, but they are not ideal for the average child. Like their sugar-sweetened counterparts, many artificially sweetened foods are simply flavored fillers such as diet sodas and candy, which provide few, if any, nutrients. Often they are cited as useful in preventing tooth decay—though such claims are erroneous; low-calorie soft drinks, for instance, are highly acidic and will dissolve dental enamel. Water should be the beverage of choice between meals.

Teenagers Make Healthy Changes, Given the Chance

THE FOLLOWING STUDY shows the real benefits of controlling the supply lines.

Consumption of sugar-sweetened drinks—sodas, sports drinks, juice drinks, sweetened iced tea, lemonade, and punch—has surged in recent decades, in step with the surge in childhood obesity. So is there a connection?

In a controlled trial at Children's Hospital in Boston, Cara Ebbeling, PhD, David Ludwig, MD, PhD, and their fellow researchers investigated the effect of decreasing sugar-sweetened beverages on body weight. "We opted to study one simple, potentially high-impact behavior, and made it easy for adolescents to replace sugary drinks with noncaloric beverages in the home," noted Ebbeling.

They enrolled 103 children ages thirteen to eighteen through a Boston area high school. The teens were offered a $100 mall gift certificate if they stuck with the six-month study (which they all did). Half the group received weekly deliveries of noncaloric beverages of their own choosing—bottled waters and artificially sweetened drinks. They were instructed on how to avoid sugar-sweetened beverages and given tips on choosing noncaloric drinks outside the home. Prompts included monthly phone calls and refrigerator magnets ("THINK BEFORE YOU DRINK"). The rest of the teens, serving as a control group, continued with their usual eating and drinking patterns. At the end of six months, the beverage delivery group had an 82 percent reduction in consumption of sugary drinks, while sugary drink intake in the control group remained unchanged.

The heavier the teen was initially, the stronger the effect on body weight. Among the heaviest one-third of teens, there was a marked decrease in body mass index (BMI) in the beverage-delivery group, and a slight increase in the control group—a group-to-group difference of almost one pound per month. Other factors affecting obesity—physical activity levels and television viewing—did not change in either group.

■ Does Sugar Affect ■ Children's Behavior?

Although some people believe sugar causes attention deficit disorder (ADD) or hyperactivity in children, results from many published studies have failed to provide any scientifically proven support for this. In situations where the investigator, the child, and the parent were unaware of the composition of the test food or capsule, refined sugar showed no effect on cognitive performance, nor did it cause or exacerbate ADD.

It is possible that a very small number of children may respond adversely to fluctuations in blood glucose levels caused by sugar. But if this is the case, any carbohydrate, including bread and potatoes, will have a similar effect.

On the whole, more evidence shows that sugar might actually have a calming effect, if it has any effect at all. Glucose or sugar can reduce the distress associated with painful medical procedures in infants. In one study, there was a reduction in crying and heart rate in infants subjected to heel pricks when they were given a sugar solution immediately prior to the procedure, compared to children who were given just water.

■ What About Fat in a Child's Diet? ■

Young children (under age two) rely on a certain amount of fat in their diet as a source of calories and should generally not be placed on a low-fat diet. A moderate amount of fat is also necessary as a source of essential fatty acids and fat-soluble vitamins. Kids need some fat—but don't go overboard. Children, like adults, should not regularly consume prepared foods that are high in saturated fat, such as cookies, cakes, pastries, ready-to-eat meals, candy, and snack foods.

■ What About Snacks? ■

Children need regular meals and snacks (at least 5–6 times per day). Young children actually can't meet their energy needs for growth and activity with just three meals. For older children, snacks provide a third to a half of their energy intake. It is therefore important that the snacks offered contribute nutrients in proportion to energy (calorie) contribution.

If you are on the go or if you find portion control helpful, prepackaged single-serving snacks can be a help. Granola bars, breakfast bars, yogurt beverages, yogurt and granola mixes, nut bars, dried fruit and nut mixes, dried fruit bars, and packages of cheese slices all fall into this category. But if it comes in a package, read the label carefully and compare brands.

And remember, kids tend to grab what's in the pantry, refrigerator, or freezer, so if you control the supply lines, they are more likely to snack right.

Healthy, portable snacks for the day

- Banana
- Small box of low-fat flavored milk
- Apple
- Granola or nut bar
- Container of low-fat yogurt
- Handful of nuts, preferably unsalted
- Handfuls of raw vegetables—e.g., carrot, red pepper, or celery sticks; fresh green beans; cucumber pieces; cherry tomatoes
- Matchbox-sized piece of cheese
- 2 tablespoons of pumpkin or sunflower seeds

For much more advice about feeding yourself and your children, see part 4, Your Guide to Low-GI Eating. We also encourage you to consult *The New Glucose Revolution Life Plan* or *The New Glucose Revolution Low GI Vegetarian Cookbook*, where you'll find dozens and dozens of family-friendly, low-GI recipes. *The Low GI Vegetarian Cookbook* also includes special menu plans for vegetarian and vegan children and teenagers.

Rising Rates of Children with Type 2 Diabetes

ACCORDING TO A report in the May 2006 issue of *Archives of Pediatrics and Adolescent Medicine*, around 39,000 teenagers between the ages of twelve and nineteen may have type 2 diabetes, and 2.8 million may have prediabetes (or **impaired fasting glucose levels**). These estimates derive from data gathered through the National Health and Nutrition Examination Survey (1999–2002) and have important implications for public health because of the high rate with which adults with prediabetes develop type 2 diabetes and the increased risk of cardiovascular disease in individuals with type 2 diabetes.

In the past, when a child was diagnosed with diabetes, the typical symptoms of weight loss, dehydration, and constant hunger and thirst made it easy to classify as type 1 (formerly known as juvenile or insulin-dependent diabetes). In recent years, a new picture has emerged.

- Instead of being thin, these children are fat.
- Instead of their bodies not making insulin, their bodies are making lots of insulin.

In the United States, most children with type 2 diabetes are being diagnosed in ethnic groups that already have a high susceptibility: African Americans, Latinos, Pacific Islanders, subcontinental Indians, and Asians. This link with ethnicity reflects a genetic susceptibility, as does a strong family history of type 2 diabetes. For example, we know it's highly likely that a child with type 2 will have at least one parent or grandparent with type 2 diabetes.

The link between type 2 diabetes in children and obesity is very strong—around 80 percent of children with type 2 are obese. So it comes as no surprise to find that the rising incidence of type 2 in young people parallels the rising incidence of overweight and obesity.

A major contributor to childhood obesity is lack of physical activity; children are not exercising nearly enough, being driven places instead of walking or bike riding, and watching television or sitting in front of computer screens instead of running around and playing vigorously. We also know that less physically active kids are more insulin resistant—another major risk factor for developing type 2.

MANAGING TYPE 2 IN CHILDREN AND TEENS

Type 2 diabetes in children is managed successfully through a combination of regular physical activity, healthy eating, and, for some young people, medication.

The aim is to:

- normalize blood glucose levels
- reduce blood fats (cholesterol and triglycerides) and blood pressure
- prevent complications

One of the key ways of achieving these goals is by managing weight. Essentially, intake of energy (calories) from food has to decrease and output of energy (physical activity) has to increase. The whole family will benefit from being healthier and fitter as a result of the diet and lifestyle changes you make to support a child with diabetes. These changes will also benefit any family members who also have diabetes or prediabetes.

Increasing energy output through physical activity is absolutely essential to manage type 2 diabetes, in both children and adults. Exercise recommendations are the same as for adults with type 2 diabetes: at least thirty minutes of some kind of physical activity most days of the week is essential. And kids (and adults) will need at least double that amount of exercise to lose weight.

Many different approaches to managing the diet of a child with type 2 diabetes are available: a weighed and measured calorie-controlled plan; simple lifestyle changes, such as including more fruit, vegetables, and whole grains in the diet; and limiting the number of treats. If your child has type 2 diabetes, you and your child should see an accredited dietitian as soon after the diagnosis as possible, to find the right approach. Keep in mind it needs to be someone you are both comfortable talking to and working with over the long haul.

FIVE PROVEN STRATEGIES FOR A HEALTHIER HOUSEHOLD DIET

1. Have regular family meals.
2. Serve a variety of healthy foods and snacks.
3. Be a role model by eating healthily yourself.
4. Involve kids in the process of food choice and preparation.
5. Avoid battles over food.

·12·

The Glycemic Index and Peak Athletic Performance

*W*hether you're a high-performance or professional athlete, or you exercise recreationally, you can benefit from learning about which foods have high and low GI values and when to eat them. For professionals and amateurs alike, it's not only the type of carbohydrate that matters, but the amount of carbohydrate is equally important. Training diets must contain sufficient carbohydrate if the GI is to make any difference at all.

■ A Diet with Sufficient Carbohydrate ■ Is Essential for Peak Athletic Performance

The reason is simple: a sufficient intake of carbohydrate when training is essential to maintain stores of muscle glycogen. As we have previously described, the carbohydrate we eat is stored in the body in the form of glycogen in the muscles and liver. A small amount of carbohydrate (about 5 grams) circulates as glucose in the blood. When you are exercising at a high intensity, your muscles rely on glycogen and glucose for fuel. Although the body can use fat when exercising at lower intensities, fat cannot provide the fuel fast enough when you are working very hard. The bigger your stores of glycogen and glucose, the longer you can go before fatigue sets in.

■

Manipulating the GI values of your diet can give you the winning edge.

■

A Low-GI Diet Increases Endurance in Athletes

ATHLETES OFTEN CONSUME high-carb foods or drinks after exercise to replace their muscle-glycogen stores as rapidly as possible—especially when they're training and competing on consecutive days. A recent study from the Nutrition Research Group at Loughborough University in the UK led by Dr. Emma Stevenson compared the effects of high- and low-GI carbohydrate recovery diets in the twenty-four hours following prolonged heavy exercise. Nine active male athletes took part in two trials. On the first day they ran for ninety minutes at 70 percent VO2 max (maximal oxygen consumption) and then ate either a high- or low-GI recovery meal, which provided them with 8 grams of carbohydrate per body mass. The next day, after an overnight fast, they ran to exhaustion. Researchers discovered that athletes who ate a low-GI diet in the twenty-four hours following prolonged running *increased* endurance capacity the next day, beyond that which was achieved after they'd eaten a high-GI carbohydrate recovery diet.

Unlike the fat stores in the body, which can release almost unlimited amounts of fatty acids, the body's carbohydrate stores are limited. They are fully depleted after two or three hours of strenuous exercise. This depletion of muscle glycogen stores is often called "hitting the wall"—essentially, a "wall of fatigue" that you can't get through. If exercise continues at the same rate, blood glucose may also drop to levels that interfere with brain function and cause disorientation and unconsciousness. Some athletes refer to this as a "hypo," and in cycling it is known as "bonking." (See chapter 8 for a fuller discussion of hypos.)

All else being equal, the eventual winner is the person with adequate carbohydrate reserves. Any good book on nutrition for athletes will tell you how to optimize your muscle glycogen stores by ingesting enough carbohydrate in your training diet—and by carbo loading on the day prior to a competition, if you're competing in a long-duration event like a marathon or triathlon. Our focus here is to provide instructions for increasing muscle glycogen as well as using the glycemic index to your advantage in any sports situation.

■ Low-GI Foods: Before a Race ■ or Other Strenuous Exercise

In some studies, low-GI foods have helped to extend endurance when eaten alone one to two hours before prolonged strenuous exercise. When a pre-event meal of lentils (low GI value) was compared with one of potatoes (high GI value), cyclists were able to continue cycling at high intensity (65 percent of their maximum capacity) for twenty minutes longer when the meal had a low GI value. Their blood glucose and insulin levels were still above fasting levels at the end of exercise, suggesting that carbohydrates were continuing to be absorbed from the small intestine even after ninety minutes of strenuous exercise. Figure 9 (see next page) shows the blood glucose levels during exercise after consumption of low- and high-GI foods.

These findings were later supported by several other research groups in the United States. Some studies, however, have not been able to show a difference between high- and low-GI foods. One explanation may be the use of different experimental protocols. Researchers who obtained a positive finding invariably used the "time to exhaustion" as the criterion for comparison, while those who showed no effect used a "time trial" (i.e., the amount of work done or distance traveled over a set time period).

Despite the fact that they were not able to show a difference in

work output between high and low foods, *all of them* showed a difference in blood glucose and insulin levels, and all of them showed differences in the ratio of carbohydrate and fat in the fuel mix. In the
high-GI trials, more carbohydrate and less fat were burned over the
course of the exercise. In theory, this could result in faster carbohydrate depletion and less time before "hitting the wall." Many athletes
choose to use low-GI foods before an event; pasta, for example, a classic low-GI food, remains a popular choice for many athletes.

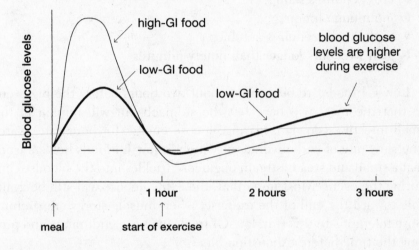

**FIGURE 8. Comparison of the effect of low- and high-GI foods on blood glucose levels dur-
ing prolonged strenuous exercise.**

Before you read any further, it's important to appreciate the *type* of
event where low-GI foods will help: specifically, it is one in which the
athlete is undertaking a very strenuous form of exercise for longer than
ninety minutes. Exercise physiologists define this by saying that the athlete is exercising at more than 65 percent of his or her maximum capacity for a prolonged period. Examples of such events include a running
or swimming marathon, a triathlon, nonstop tennis competition, or a
soccer game (depending on the player's position). In some forms of
recreation, such as cross-country skiing and mountain climbing, an athlete may also benefit from low-GI foods. In some occupations that
require prolonged strenuous activity for hours and hours (such as police
rescue or forest firefighting), low-GI foods may also be beneficial.

■ Events in Which the Glycemic Index ■ May Give You the Edge

- ▶ running marathon
- ▶ swimming marathon
- ▶ triathlon
- ▶ nonstop tennis competition
- ▶ soccer game (depending on the player's position)
- ▶ cross-country skiing
- ▶ mountain climbing
- ▶ prolonged strenuous aerobics
- ▶ gym workouts longer than ninety minutes

Low-GI foods are best eaten about two hours before the big event so that the meal will have left the stomach but will remain in the small intestine, slowly releasing glucose energy, for hours afterward. The slow rate of carbohydrate digestion in low-GI foods helps ensure that a small and steady stream of glucose trickles into the bloodstream during the event. Most important, the extra glucose will still be available toward the end of the exercise, when muscle stores are running close to empty. In this way, low-GI foods increase endurance and prolong the time before exhaustion hits.

■ The Pre-Event Meal ■

How much should I eat before the event? Consume at least 1 gram of carbohydrate for every 2 pounds of body weight (i.e., 55 grams of carbohydrate if you weigh 110 pounds or 90 grams of carbohydrate if you weigh 180 pounds).

How soon before? A good starting point is about two hours before the event. You should experiment to determine the timing that works best for you. You will find the amounts of carbohydrate in a nominal serving of food (along with their GI values and glycemic load) in the tables in part 5 of this book.

In any sports context, it's critical to select low-GI foods that do not cause gastrointestinal discomfort (stomach cramps and/or flatulence).

Some low-GI foods—such as legumes, which are high in fiber or indigestible sugars—may produce symptoms in people not used to eating large amounts of them. The good news, though, is that you have many low-fiber, low-GI choices, including pasta, noodles, and basmati rice.

■ High-GI Foods ■
During and After a Race or Strenuous Exercise

Scientific evidence indicates that there are times when high-GI foods are preferable—specifically, during and after events. This is because high-GI foods are absorbed faster and stimulate more insulin, the hormone responsible for getting glucose back into the muscles for either immediate or future use.

The GI Values of Sports Drinks and Sports Bars

DRINKS	GI
GatorLode (orange)	100
Gatorade (orange)	78
XLR8 (orange)	68
Powerade (orange)	65
Cytomax (orange)	62
AllSport (orange)	53
BARS	**GI**
Clif bar (cookies & cream)	101
PowerBar (chocolate)	56
MET-Rx bar (vanilla)	74

During the event. High-GI foods should be used during events lasting longer than ninety minutes. This form of carbohydrate is rapidly released into the bloodstream and ensures that glucose is available for oxidation in the muscle cells. Sports drinks are ideal during the race because they replace electrolytes as well as water. Although bananas have a GI of only 55, they remain a popular choice because they are easy to eat and can help you to fill the hunger void that may occur in longer events. If you want to go for a high-GI, fast-energy source, try jelly beans (GI = 80) or another form of high-glucose candy. Consume 30 to 60 grams of carbohydrate per hour during the event.

After the event (recovery). In some competitive sports, athletes compete on consecutive days, and glycogen stores need to be restored rapidly. In this case, it's important to restock the glycogen store in the muscles as quickly as possible after the event. High-GI foods are best in this situation. Muscles are more sensitive to glucose in the bloodstream in the first hour after exercise, so a concerted effort should be made to get as many high-GI foods in as soon as possible.

Ideal foods include most of the sports drinks on the market (which replace both water and electrolyte losses), or high-GI rice (e.g., jasmine), breads, and breakfast cereals such as cornflakes and Rice Krispies. Potatoes cooked without fat are a good choice, too, but they tend to be dense and filling, which can make it hard to eat lots of them. It is important to remember that athletes need to concentrate on consuming a balanced diet in the recovery period—one that provides enough carbohydrate to meet their needs. Using high-GI carbs at this time helps to ensure that recovery is not delayed.

A word about alcohol: While most alcohol has no GI value (beer is the exception; its GI is 66, as we explain on pages 157–158), it's problematic because it may interfere with glycogen resynthesis and lower blood glucose levels, sometimes to dangerous levels. Keep alcohol intake moderate—no more than one or two drinks per day, and try to have two alcohol-free days a week. An average drink is equivalent to one glass of wine (5 ounces), one 12-ounce bottle of beer, or 1½ ounces of liquor. (And a reminder: beer is not a good source of carbohydrate; a 12-ounce bottle of beer contains about 11 to 13 grams of carbohydrate; a can of light beer, by contrast, has 3 to 6 grams.)

∎

THE BASIC RECOVERY FORMULA: Aim to ingest about 1 gram of carbohydrate per 2 pounds of body weight every 2 hours after exercise.

∎

A word about serving size. Athletes with high energy expenditure need to choose large portions (for instance, on race days, riders in the Tour de France take in 6,000–7,000 calories). Of course, there will be times when you don't feel like eating a big meal of rice or pasta, so at those times sports drinks and soft drinks are a good option. Choose what you can tolerate and what's easy and practical for you to bring or buy. The main point is to make sure you eat and drink carbohydrate soon after the exercise session.

To Maximize Glycogen
Replenishment after a Race or Strenuous Exercise

- Ingest carbohydrate as soon as you can after the event, and maintain an adequate carbohydrate intake for the next 24 hours.
- Choose high-GI foods during your replenishment phase.
- Avoid alcohol.

■ The Training Diet and Carb Loading ■

It's not just your pre- and post-event meals that influence your performance. Consuming enough carbohydrate every day will help you reach peak performance. The GI value of the carbohydrate is not the issue here—only the amount of carbohydrate. Carbohydrate stores need to be replenished after each training session, not just after a race. If you train on a number of days per week, make sure you consume enough carbohydrate throughout the week.

■ How to Choose a High-Carbohydrate Diet ■

Dietary advice directed at the general public needs to be modified for serious athletes, whether professionals or amateurs. Athletes usually have far greater energy needs—possibly double that of someone who has a sedentary office job. Athletes with high energy needs may struggle

Is Your Diet Fit for Peak Performance?

TAKE THE DIET-FITNESS quiz below and see how well you score. It's a good idea to use this quiz regularly to pick up on areas where you may need to improve your diet.

1. CIRCLE YOUR ANSWER.

- I eat at least 3 meals a day with no longer than 5 hours in between.   Yes/No

EATING PATTERNS

Carbohydrate checker

- I eat at least 4 slices of bread each day (1 roll = 2 slices of bread).   Yes/No
- I eat at least 1 cup of breakfast cereal each day or an extra slice of bread.   Yes/No
- I usually eat 2 or more pieces of fruit each day.   Yes/No
- I eat at least 3 different vegetables or have a salad most days.   Yes/No
- I include carbohydrate like pasta, rice, and potatoes in my diet each day.   Yes/No

Protein checker

- I eat at least 1 and usually 2 servings of meat or meat alternatives (poultry, seafood, eggs, dried peas/beans, or nuts) each day.   Yes/No

Fat checker

- I spread butter or margarine thinly on bread or use none at all.   Yes/No
- I eat fried food no more than once per week.   Yes/No
- I use polyunsaturated or monounsaturated oil (canola or olive) for cooking (circle yes if you never fry in oil or fat).   Yes/No
- I avoid oil-based dressings on salads.   Yes/No
- I use reduced-fat or low-fat dairy products.   Yes/No
- I cut the fat off meat and take the skin off chicken.   Yes/No

- I eat fatty snacks such as chocolate, chips, Yes/No
  cookies, or rich desserts/cakes, etc. no more
  than twice a week.
- I eat fast or take-out food no more than once per week. Yes/No

Iron checker
- I eat lean red meat at least 3 times per week Yes/No
  or 2 servings of white meat daily or, for vegetarians,
  include at least 1–2 cups of dried peas and beans
  (e.g., lentils, soy beans, chickpeas) daily.
- I include a vitamin C source with meals Yes/No
  based on bread, cereals, fruits, and vegetables
  to assist the iron absorption in these "plant"
  sources of iron.

Calcium checker
- I eat at least 3 servings of dairy food or Yes/No
  soy milk alternative each day (1 serving = 8 oz
  milk or fortified soy milk; 1 slice (1½ oz)
  hard cheese; 8 oz yogurt).

Fluids
- I drink fluids regularly before, during, and Yes/No
  after exercise.

Alcohol
- When I drink alcohol, I would mostly drink no more Yes/No
  than is recommended for the safe drunk-driving limit
  (circle yes if you don't drink alcohol).

2. SCORE 1 POINT FOR EVERY "YES" ANSWER

Scoring scale

18–20 Excellent	15–17 Room for improvement
12–14 Just made it	0–12 Poor

Note: Very active people will need to eat more breads, cereals, and
fruit than on this quiz, but to stay healthy no one should be eating less.

with consuming enough carbohydrate, as the "bulk" of these foods may make it difficult to consume enough. For example, a 75-gram carbohydrate portion of potatoes is equal to more than a pound of potatoes—about four normal servings. Most people (even a hungry athlete) simply can't eat that much at a time. On the other hand, white bread is easier to eat in large amounts. A 75-gram carbohydrate portion of white bread is only five slices. White rice and pasta are also nutritious sources of carbohydrate that deliver a substantial amount without being too bulky. In some cases athletes may need to supplement their carbohydrate intake with very-low-bulk carbohydrate sources. Sports drinks (e.g., Gatorade, Powerade) can be very convenient to support needs during a training session. There also may be a little room for foods that you might have believed were not so good for you, like soft drinks, candy, honey, sugar, flavored milk, and ice cream. These provide carbohydrate in an energy-dense form that can be used to supplement needs.

Can a High-GI Diet Be Harmful to Athletes?

THE SHORT ANSWER is: we don't think so. By virtue of their high activity levels, athletes have optimal insulin sensitivity. When they eat high-carbohydrate, high-GI foods, blood glucose and insulin levels rise far less in them than in the average person. As a result, their bodies are not exposed to the dangerous levels that produce disease in sedentary, insulin-resistant individuals.

PART 3

Questions & Answers

Frequently asked questions about

the glycemic index, answered

▪13▪

Frequently Asked Questions About the Glycemic Index, Answered

*S*ince the first edition of this book was published, we've heard from thousands of readers from all over the world asking us to clarify or elaborate on many different aspects of the GI, carbohydrates, and diet. The most frequently asked of those questions are here, as well as those that we think are of the most interest to the widest array of readers.

The Q&A's are grouped into the following six subject categories:

- ▸ GI values of specific foods and food groups
- ▸ Sugar and starch
- ▸ GI and mixed meals, portion sizes, and the myth of diet restriction
- ▸ GI and diabetes
- ▸ GI, blood glucose, and other metabolic processes
- ▸ Advanced Q&A's for clinicians, researchers, and the very curious

We encourage you to write to us if your questions aren't answered here or elsewhere in this book (or in others in our series—see page iv). Send your questions to gifeedback@gmail.com.

■ Q&A's about GI Values of Specific Foods ■ and Food Groups

High, Medium, or Low GI . . .

- A high GI value is 70 or more.
- A medium/moderate GI value is 56–69 inclusive.
- A low GI value is 55 or less.

What's the GI of a caffè latte and a cappuccino?

Most coffee-and-milk drinks will have a low GI and won't be too highly caloric, so long as you don't sweeten them with more than a teaspoon or so of sugar and you say no to flavored syrups lined up on the counter. In fact, a caffè latte, cappuccino, or café au lait can be an easy way to help you get your 2 to 3 daily servings of dairy foods. Regular or skim milk has a low GI (27–34)—a function of the moderate glycemic effect of its sugar (lactose) plus milk protein, which forms a soft curd in the stomach and slows down stomach emptying. (All this said, it's worth noting that some coffee drinks available at coffee shops can be very highly caloric—for instance, many drinks similar to Coffe Whips or Frappuccinos at coffee chains clock in north of 400–500 calories—some even have as many as 730 calories. The more complicated your coffee drink, the greater the chance that it is, in fact, highly caloric.)

Regular whole milk is high in saturated fat, but the wide range of reduced-fat milks—including skim, 1%, and 2%—are readily available alternatives. If you prefer soy milk (GI = 36–45, for reduced fat), make sure you opt for calcium-fortified *and* reduced fat. We don't recommend rice milk as a suitable substitute; it has a high GI (79).

How much milk are you getting with your coffee? Well, to some extent it depends on the barista and where you buy it. But here are some standard definitions:

▶ **Cappuccino** is traditionally equal parts espresso, steamed milk, and frothed milk.

▶ **Café au lait** is similar except it is generally made with brewed coffee instead of espresso in a ratio of 1:1 milk to coffee.

▶ **Caffè latte** is a single shot of espresso with steamed milk— approximately a 3:1 ratio of milk to coffee.

Some soft drinks have a low GI.
How often should children be allowed them?

Sweetened drinks (including sodas and sweetened juices), even if they have a low GI, are definitely not an everyday beverage. Here's why: liquid calories are a little stealthier than most, in that they tend to sneak past the satiety center in your brain, which would normally help to stop you from overeating. This isn't to say that everyone should avoid full-strength soft drinks all the time, but to keep on the healthy diet food–frequency scale, consumption ought to rank as "occasional" (or even "keep for a treat" if you're trying to lose weight)—and definitely not be consumed every day.

If consumption figures are any indication, an increase in sugar-sweetened soft drinks and juices is contributing to our child obesity problem. Not only have fatter children been found to have higher consumption, but overall, our children are drinking more of these sweetened drinks than their parents did when they were children. And of course the increase in serving size from the old-fashioned 8 oz (240 ml) to the widely available 17 oz (500 ml) "buddy" size doesn't help. Soft drinks aren't the only problem, either. Too much fruit juice, sweetened or unsweetened, is an easy way for us to gulp down extra calories.

Potatoes, one of my favorite foods, have high GI values.
Does this mean I have to avoid them?

First of all, you need not say "no" to potatoes altogether just because they may have a high GI. They are fat free (when you don't fry them), nutrient rich, and filling. Not every food you eat has to have a low GI. Enjoy them, but in moderation.

Second, look for lower-GI varieties, or serve them in a way that reduces the glycemic response. University of Toronto researchers found that the GI of potatoes ranged from 65 to 88, depending on the variety and cooking method. Precooking and reheating potatoes or consuming cold cooked potatoes (such as potato salad) reduced the glycemic response. Freshly cooked and mashed potatoes had the highest GI. And researchers at Sweden's University of Lund found that preparing potatoes the day before and serving them cold as potato salad with vinegar or a vinaigrette dressing can lower the GI.

Third, remember that potatoes are a relative newcomer to the western dinner plate. Athough the Spanish brought them back to Europe from South America in the mid-sixteenth century, people regarded them with suspicion, as fit only for animals. They didn't become a regular part of the European diet until the late eighteenth century and into the nineteenth century, when they replaced traditional whole-grain staples such as wheat, barley, rye, and oats, which have much lower GI values. So look back for a healthy future and add variety to your meals by enjoying whole grains, legumes, pasta, noodles, and basmati rice on a regular basis—and potatoes occasionally. And keep those portions moderate. You'll reduce the overall GI and GL of your diet and your risk of chronic disease.

> **Low-GI cooking tip:** (We're asked about potatoes so often, we're repeating this tip, which also appeared earlier): If potatoes are your favorite food, don't cut them out—instead, eat them in moderation, cut your usual portion in half and add a lower GI accompaniment like sweet corn, or cook them ahead of time—then cool and reheat before eating (which lowers the GI). Steam small new potatoes (with their skin for added nutrients), or bake a potato and add a tasty, low-GI topping— again, sweet corn, beans, or chickpeas. If you love mashed potatoes, substitute half the potato with white beans such as cannellini. Boiled potatoes or a simple potato salad made with a vinaigrette dressing have a lower GI and are a much better choice for weight control than French fries or potato chips, which are far higher in fat and calories.

What's the GI of beef, chicken, fish, eggs, nuts, and avocados? (I don't see these foods in some GI lists.)

These foods contain no carbohydrates or so little that their GI can't be tested according to the standard methodology. Essentially, these types of foods, when eaten alone, won't have much effect on your blood glucose levels. Because we're constantly asked about them, we now include these foods in the tables in part 5, and have given them a GI value of 0. Likewise, the glycemic load of these foods is 0.

Why is there no GI for blueberries, blackberries, and raspberries?

Most berries have so little carbohydrate it's difficult to test their GI (except for strawberries: GI = 40). Berries' low carbohydrate content means their glycemic load will be low, so you can enjoy them by the bowlful. They are a good source of vitamin C and fiber; some berries also supply small amounts of folate and such essential minerals as potassium, iron, calcium, magnesium, and phosphorus. Eat them fresh, add them to fruit salads and smoothies, use them in a delicious dessert, decorate cakes with them, or make them into jams, fruit spreads, and sauces.

As for fresh strawberries, they are rich in vitamin C, potassium, folate, fiber, and protective antioxidants. Because a typical serving size has very little impact on blood glucose levels, people with diabetes can eat them freely (but hold the cream!). *A word of warning*: Don't eat too many strawberries in a single day; they can have diuretic and laxative effects if you overdo it.

Does the GI increase with serving size?
If I eat twice as much, does the GI double?

The GI always remains the same, even if you double the amount of carbohydrate in your meal. This is because the GI is a relative ranking that compares one source of carbohydrate with another, per gram of carbohydrate. But if you double the amount of food you eat, you can expect to see a higher blood glucose response—that is, your glucose levels will reach a higher peak and take longer to return to baseline compared with a normal serving size. This is where GL—a measure of the glycemic potency of foods per average serving—comes in handy, because it puts together both the amount of carbohydrate you eat and its GI to help predict how much a serving of food will raise blood glucose. (See page 16 for our fuller discussion of GL.)

What's the GI of alcoholic beverages?

Generally, alcoholic beverages contain very little carbohydrate. Most wines and spirits contain virtually none; regular beer contains around 10 to 13 grams of carbohydrate per 12-oz bottle; stout around

14 grams of carbohydrate per 12-oz bottle, while a light beer has from 3 to 6 grams of carbohydrate per serving (again, a 12-oz bottle). A can of regular (not diet) soda, on the other hand, has between 35 and 45 grams of carbohydrate.

Because beer has so little carbohydrate, it's difficult to test its GI—which is why we haven't tested many brands of beer; and why we listed its GI and GL as 0 in earlier editions of this book and others in our series. But eventually we decided that the valid way to test beer would be by comparing responses to a 10-gram carbohydrate portion of beer (about 300 mL) with a 10-gram carbohydrate portion of glucose (as we explain on pages 10–11, in chapter 2, in GI testing a 50-gram carbohydrate portion is normally used). In this test, beer's GI is 66. Its glycemic load can be calculated as follows: $66 \times 10 \div 100 = 6.6$ (or, rounded up, GL = 7).

Thus, beer will raise glucose levels a little, but not a lot. If you drink beer in large volumes (not a good idea anyway, from an overall health perspective), then you could expect it to have a significant effect on blood glucose.

Why do most varieties of rice have such a high GI value?

It's true, most varieties of rice are high GI—over 70 is typical, even in imported varieties from Thailand and brown rice. The reason can be traced back to the state of gelatinization of the starch in the cooked grains (see page 20). Despite rice's "whole-grain" nature, complete gelatinization takes place during cooking—meaning millions of microscopic cracks and fissures in the grains allow water to penetrate right to the middle of the grain during cooking, allowing the starch granules to swell and the starch to hydrate.

Nonetheless, some varieties of white rice, such as basmati, have substantially lower GI values. The reason: they have more amylose starch, which resists gelatinization. If you are a big rice eater, we recommend choosing basmati or Uncle Ben's converted, or, alternatively, rice noodles (rice vermicelli is low GI). If you like sushi, you're also in luck. The vinegar used in making sushi as well as in nori (seaweed) helps to lower sushi's GI to 48.

I have read in some GI lists that fresh coconut is low GI. Is this true?
Coconut does not seem to be on your list.

Coconut is a nut (not a fruit), and it has not been GI tested. It contains very little carbohydrate per serving (just 1 gram in a 15-gram portion), and it is virtually impossible to GI test. But it is high in fat (5 gram in a 15-gram portion), and the fat it contains is nearly 90 percent saturated. So when cooking, use very small amounts of coconut milk, flaked (desiccated) coconut, or other products made from coconut.

Why has the GI value of carrots changed from 92 to 41?

When carrots were first tested in 1981, their GI was 92, but only five people were included in the study, and the variation among them was huge. This was in the early days of GI testing, and the reference food was tested only once. When carrots were assessed more recently, ten people were included, the reference food was tested twice, and a mean value of 41 was obtained, with narrow variation. It was clear that this result was more accurate and that the other value should be ignored. Unfortunately, one of the most repeated criticisms of the GI approach was the fact that carrots were being excluded from diets simply because of their high GI. This demonstrates the need for reliable, standardized methodology for GI testing. It is also another case for not using the GI in isolation when creating a healthy diet plan.

What's the GI of cornstarch?

We're often asked about the GI of such thickeners as arrowroot, cornstarch, kudzu root powder, and instant tapioca. These starchy powders thicken sauces, soups, and pie fillings without adding fat or going lumpy. All you do is mix about a tablespoon of cornstarch in a tablespoon of water, whisk that into the liquid you are thickening, and cook for about a minute, stirring constantly to remove the slightly starchy flavor. These proportions will make about 1 cup (8 oz.) of a medium-thick sauce.

As far as we know, none of these thickeners has been GI tested (at least we haven't seen any published results). However, you are using only very small amounts diluted in a cup or more of liquid or pie filling. So the GI of the recipe really depends on what you're making.

> **Low-GI cooking tip:** Here are some alternative ideas for thickening sauces and soups:
>
> - **Sauces:** Simply reducing the sauce will thicken it and intensify the flavor.
> - **Soups:** For vegetable soups, using a blender, food processor, or food mill, purée some of the cooked vegetables, then stir them back into the soup to thicken. Adding grated starchy vegetables like sweet potato or yams will also thicken a vegetable soup; or stale, well-crumbled bread crumbs (sourdough or grainy, of course) to a mushroom soup. For a creamy soup, you can stir in a little light evaporated milk or low-fat yogurt. Puréed cooked or canned white beans will also thicken a vegetable soup.

A high-fat food may have a low GI. Doesn't this make these foods sound healthful, even when they're not?

It can—especially if the fat that the food contains is saturated. That's why it's important to think about all of the different nutritional qualities of a food, and not only its GI.

For example, potato chips and French fries are lower GI than baked potatoes. Corn chips are lower GI than sweet corn. The reason: large amounts of fat in food tend to slow the rate of stomach emptying and therefore the rate at which foods are digested. Yet the saturated fat in these foods makes them less healthful and contributes to a greatly increased risk of heart disease.

If we were to weigh the health benefits of a high-GI but low-fat food (e.g., mashed potatoes) versus one high in saturated fat but low GI (e.g., some cookies), then we vote for the potatoes. Again, the GI was never meant to be the sole determinant of what foods you choose to eat. Instead, it's essential to base your food choices on the overall nutrient content of a food, including fiber, fat, and salt.

Another important point to stress here: not all high-fat foods are unhealthy. Foods that contain heart-healthy fats—avocados, nuts, and legumes—are excellent foods. Foods that contain saturated fats, even if they're low GI—such as full-fat dairy products, cakes, and cookies—are not as healthy. Save them for special occasions.

Why are many high-fiber foods high GI?

Dietary fiber is not one chemical constituent; rather, it's composed of many different sorts of molecules. As we explained in chapter 2 (see "The Effect of Fiber on the Glycemic Index," page 25, fiber can be divided into soluble and insoluble types. Soluble fiber is often viscous (thick and jellylike) in solution and remains viscous even in the small intestine. It slows down digestion, making it harder for enzymes to digest the food. Foods with more soluble fiber, like apples, oats, and legumes, are low GI as a result. Insoluble fiber, on the other hand, is not viscous and doesn't slow digestion, especially if it's finely milled. This is why whole-grain bread and white bread have similar GIs, and why brown pasta and brown rice have values similar to those of their white counterparts.

I'm an avid cook, and I often make my own bread, pancakes, muffins, cookies, and other baked goods. Which flours, if any, are low GI? Chickpea flour (baisen) appears to be low GI. What about soy flour? I'm guessing that whole-wheat flour probably isn't any better than white, judging by the results on commercial breads.

To date there are no GI values for any refined flours—whether those refined from wheat, soy, or other grains. This is because the GI rating of a food must be determined physiologically (in real people). So far we haven't had volunteers willing to consume 50-gram portions of flour on three occasions! What we do know, however, is that bakery products such as scones, cakes, biscuits, doughnuts, and pastries made from highly refined flour, whether white or whole wheat, are quickly digested and absorbed.

With your own baking, try to increase the soluble fiber content by partially replacing flour with oat bran, rice bran, or rolled oats. You can also increase the bulkiness of your baked goods by adding dried fruit, nuts, muesli, All-Bran, or unprocessed bran. The recipes in part 4 of this book include a variety of low- and moderate-GI baked goods.

While you will benefit from eating low-GI carbs at each meal, you don't have to avoid all high-GI foods. And by combining high-GI baked goods with protein foods and low-GI carbs, such as fruit, many vegetables, or legumes, the overall GI value will be medium.

Will GI values ever be included on food labels?

Food manufacturers are increasingly interested in having the GI of their products measured—in fact, some are already testing for research purposes only and consequently withholding the data; others are going so far as to include the GI on labels. As more and more research highlights the benefits of low-GI foods, consumers and dietitians alike are asking food companies and diabetes organizations for GI data. The GI symbol ©, a trademark of the University of Sydney in Australia and in other countries (including the United States), is a public health initiative that provides consumers with a credible signpost to healthier food choices using the internationally recognized benefits of GI and sound nutrition. The GI symbol on a food package indicates that that food has been *properly* GI tested (in real people, not in a test tube) and also makes a positive contribution to nutrition. More information about the program can be found at www.gisymbol.com.

When I don't see GI information on a food product, can I estimate a food's GI by looking at the ingredients or the nutrition label?

A packaged food's Nutrition Facts panel will tell you the carbohydrate content, but it won't indicate the GI of that food. If it contains at least 10 grams of carbohydrates per serving, you can be sure it will have at least some effect on your blood glucose concentration—but there's no way of telling whether it will be a little or a lot. Similarly, you can't estimate the GI of a food by looking at its ingredient list, because it won't tell you the final state of the starches in the food—which ultimately determine GI value.

That said, we can make some generalizations about the GI of different food categories that you can keep in mind when choosing foods that haven't been GI tested. Legumes, for example, have some of the lowest GI values. Most pasta and noodle products tend to be low-GI foods (a fact that seems to surprise many—but again, it comes down to the way these products are made). Most fresh fruits are low GI, as are carbohydrate-rich dairy foods like milk, yogurt, ice cream, pudding, and custard. In contrast, most bread, bakery products, rice, and cereals are high GI, although those that are less processed will be lower GI. As we mentioned above, protein-rich foods—cheese, meat, eggs, and poultry—don't have measurable GI values, because they contain little if any carbohydrates. The same is true for salad vegetables. The most comprehensive list of GI values now available appears in the tables in part 5.

Should I add up the GI each day?

No. In some of the earliest editions of our books, we included sample menus and calculated an estimated GI for the day. As our understanding of the GI grew, and we heard from our readers and talked to our clients, we realized how unnecessary, and even misleading, this was. A food's GI can be altered by the way it is processed or cooked, so we don't believe it is possible to calculate a precise GI for recipes or to predict the GI of a menu for the whole day. That's why we now prefer in most circumstances simply to categorize foods as low, medium, or high GI. We have also found that many people who substitute low-GI for high-GI foods in their everyday meals and snacks reduce the overall GI of their diet, gain better blood glucose control, and lose weight. (For more advice on substituting low-GI for high GI foods, see "This for That" on pages 80–81 in chapter 6.)

■ Q&A's about Sugar and Starch ■

Is there a difference between naturally occurring sugars and refined sugar?

Naturally occurring sugars are those found in milk and other dairy products and fruits and vegetables, including their juices. Refined sugar means added sugar, table sugar, honey, maple syrup, or corn syrup. Both sources include varying amounts of sucrose, glucose, fructose, and lactose. Some nutritionists make a distinction between them, because natural sugars are usually accompanied by micronutrients such as vitamin C.

The rate of digestion and absorption of naturally occurring sugars is no different, on average, from that of refined sugars. There is, however, wide variation within food groups, depending on the food. The GI of fruits varies, from 25 for grapefruit to 76 for watermelon. Similarly, among the foods containing refined sugar, some are low-GI, some high. The GI of sweetened, low-fat yogurt is only 26 to 28, while a Milky Way bar (a Mars bar in Canada) has a GI of 62 (lower than bread).

Why do nutritionists still recommend starchy foods over sugary foods?

Sugar has an image problem that stems largely from research with rodents using unrealistic amounts of pure sugar. It's also seen as a source of "empty calories" (energy without vitamins or minerals) and concentrated energy. But much of the criticism doesn't stand up to actual research findings.

Most starchy foods have the same energy density as sugary foods (see "Energy Density—Key Things to Know," on page 70), and even a soft drink has the same calorie content per gram as an apple. Starchy foods, such as whole-grain cereals, can be excellent sources of vitamins, minerals, and fiber, but some pure forms of starch and modified starches are added to foods that are "empty calories." So there really isn't a big difference between sugars and starches, either in nutritional terms or in terms of the glycemic index. Our advice is to use sugar to your advantage by adding it to nutritious foods (such as brown sugar in oatmeal, honey in tea, or jam on bread) to make them taste even better.

■ Q&A's About the GI and Mixed Meals, ■ Portion Sizes, and the Myth of Diet Restriction

Can you use the glycemic index to predict the effect of a meal containing a mixture of foods with very different GI values?

Yes, the GI can predict the relative effects of different mixed meals containing foods with very different GI values. In a major study we published in the June 2006 edition of the *American Journal of Clinical Nutrition*, we found that the GI works just as predictably whether people eat a single portion of one item, or a normal meal. (See also "Can the GI Be Applied to the Meals You Eat Each Day?" on pages 14–15).

What size portion does a food's GI refer to? For example, the GI of
bananas is 55. Does this correspond to one banana—and if so, is it
for a large banana or a small one?

A food's GI value doesn't refer to a specific quantity of food;
instead, it's a measure that reflects the quality of the carbohydrate
in that food—specifically, its ability to raise blood glucose levels, no
matter what the portion size. So for your example this would mean
that 52 is the GI for one banana, small or large. The glycemic load
(GL) takes into account both the quantity and quality of carbohydrate (see pages 16–17).

Opponents of the low-GI approach say that low-GI diets are too
restrictive, that they narrow the range of foods that can be eaten. Is
this true?

It's absolutely a myth that you have to narrow the range of foods
you eat on a low-GI diet. In fact, most people who take a low-GI
approach to eating say the exact opposite: unlike many other diet
plans, the glycemic index has actually *expanded* their range of
foods, because they've been encouraged to try things they have
never eaten before (e.g., Indian dals, Asian noodles, lentil soups).
Plus, they say they're relieved to finally have "permission" to consume foods containing sugar, such as jams and ice cream.

The idea that all low-GI foods are high in fiber and not very tasty
is also a myth. All-Bran and chickpeas may not be everyone's
favorite foods, but many people enjoy low-GI foods like pasta, oats,
whole grains, legumes, and a huge variety of fruits and vegetables.
For delicious, low-GI menu ideas, see part 4 of this book.

I haven't been able to find a reference to what GI number a person
should shoot for when trying to diet. Is there a formula, such as "take
goal weight, multiply by age, divide by activity level"?

The simple answer is: no, there's no formula. You don't need to
add up the GI each day. In fact there's no counting at all as there
is with calories. The basic technique for eating the low GI way is
simply "This for That"—swapping the high-GI carbs in your diet for
low-GI foods. This could mean eating oatmeal at breakfast instead
of a high-GI cold breakfast cereal, low-GI bread instead of normal
white or whole-wheat bread, or sparkling apple juice in place of a

soft drink. So, what you need to "shoot for" is identifying the high-GI carbs in your current diet and swapping them for some quality low-GI carbs. We've found that many people who do just this reduce the overall GI of their diet, gain better blood glucose control, and lose weight.

Do I need to eat low-GI foods at every meal in order to benefit from a low-GI diet?

Not necessarily. The good news: The effect of a low-GI food carries over to the next meal, reducing the glycemic impact of higher-GI foods. This applies to a breakfast eaten after a low-GI dinner the previous evening. It also applies to lunch eaten after a low-GI breakfast. This unexpected beneficial effect of low-GI meals is called the "second meal" effect. Don't take this too far, however; on the whole, we recommend that you aim for at least one low-GI food per meal.

I have been following a low-GI diet for years to combat hypoglycemia, and I've been very happy with the results—more even energy levels and easy weight maintenance. I am about to introduce my baby to solids and have been advised to start with rice cereal. I worry about giving my baby rice cereal as her first food, especially since I (and most of my family) are so focused on eating low-GI. What is the current guidance on GI for babies and young children?

Chapter 11, Children and the Glycemic Index, gives our full thinking and recommendations with regard to children and the GI. Regarding rice cereal specifically, Dr. Heather Gilbertson, a dietitian and educator with many years' experience in management of children with diabetes, and coauthor of another of our books, *The New Glucose Revolution Guide to Healthy Kids*, advises: "Introduction of rice cereal for infants with hypoglycemia should not cause any problems. I would generally recommend mixing it with expressed breast milk, to modify the GI effect. Rice cereal is an important introductory food for babies, as it is iron-fortified. Infants need additional iron intake at six months of age to meet their requirements. The main key to managing infant hypoglycemia is to ensure [that] the baby has a regular intake of carbohydrate throughout the day (frequent feedings/meals and snacks) and avoids long periods of fasting. Foods high in added or natural sugars (fruit juices) should also be avoided, as these may aggravate the hypoglycemia.

"Deliberately avoiding or limiting carbohydrate-containing foods will also cause the blood glucose levels to drop low in an infant with a diagnosed hypoglycemic disorder. Mothers also need to encourage their babies to try a wide range of tastes and textures of the fruit and vegetable variety (focusing on either low-GI or a combination of low with high to modify the effect). As children get older, mothers can introduce dairy foods, which all have a low-GI, and other breads and cereals. Any parent who has a child with a hypoglycemic endocrine disorder should seek out individual professional nutritional advice from their local pediatric dietitian." (See page 48 on how to find a dietitian.)

Is there a GI plan for nursing mothers?

Joanna McMillan-Price, our coauthor of *The Low GI Diet Revolution* and *The Low GI Diet Revolution Cookbook*, and herself a recent mother who is breast-feeding and trying to get back into shape, advises, "A low-GI diet is ideal for while you are breast-feeding, which requires a lot of energy—and, theoretically, this additional energy comes from the body fat we laid down during pregnancy. Of course, in reality it doesn't all get used up, and most of us have to make a concerted effort to work off the baby weight. To do this, though, it is important that you don't go on a low-calorie diet or any sort of extreme measure.

"Since breast-feeding tends to increase your appetite (the body's way of ensuring you have the energy required to produce milk), this is good news—as staying on such a [low-calorie] diet would be a nightmare. This is what makes the low-GI approach so successful—you can forget about trying to count calories or even your portions of food. Make low-GI foods the mainstay of your meals, and you can trust your appetite and eat to satisfaction while you are breast-feeding. Also, get back to some exercise—even if it's just a daily walk with the stroller. You should then find that the weight slowly starts to shift—but, realistically, give yourself at least that first six months to get back to your pre-pregnancy weight."

▪ Q&A's About the GI and Diabetes ▪

Does sugar cause diabetes?

No. There is absolute consensus that sugar in food does not cause diabetes. Type 1 diabetes (insulin-dependent diabetes) is an autoimmune condition triggered by unknown environmental factors, such as viruses. Type 2 diabetes (non-insulin-dependent diabetes) is strongly inherited, but lifestyle factors, such as lack of exercise and being overweight, increase the risk of developing it. In the past, when the dietary treatment of diabetes involved strict avoidance of sugar, many people wrongly believed that sugar was in some way implicated as a cause of the disease. While sugar is off the hook, high-GI foods are not. Research at Harvard University has shown that high-GI diets increase the risk of developing both type 2 diabetes and heart disease.

Why are people with diabetes now allowed some sugar in their diet?

For a long time, people with diabetes were advised to avoid all sugar. That's because health-care professionals were taught that simple sugars were solely responsible for high blood glucose levels. But research has proved that people with diabetes can eat the same amount of sugar as the average person—without compromising diabetes control.

It's important, however, to remember that "empty calories"—whatever the source, be it sugar, starch, fat, or alcohol—won't keep your body operating optimally. The now clichéd expression "moderation in all things" has withstood the test of time for obvious reasons. We advise that you get no more than 10 percent of your total daily calories from sugar (which translates into about 3 tablespoons of sugar a day for women and about 4½ tablespoons for men). Keep in mind that this refers not only to the sugar you add to coffee or cereal but also to the sugar already contained in the foods you eat—soda, cakes, cookies, ice cream, yogurt, and so on.

Can GI values obtained from tests on healthy people be applied to people with diabetes?

Yes. Several studies show a strong correlation between values obtained in healthy people and people with diabetes (type 1 and type 2). By its very nature, GI testing takes into account differences in glucose tolerance between people. High-GI foods are still digested quickly, and low-GI foods are still digested slowly. Some people with diabetes have *gastroparesis*, a disorder in which the emptying of the stomach slows down. (People with diabetes involved with GI testing are usually screened to check that they don't have gastroparesis.) The ranking of foods according to their GI values is still applicable.

Some nonsalad vegetables, such as pumpkin, appear to have a high GI value. Does this mean people with diabetes shouldn't eat them?

Definitely not. Unlike potatoes and cereal products, these vegetables are very low in carbohydrate. So despite their high GI, their glycemic load (GI × carbohydrate per serving divided by 100) is low. Other low-carbohydrate vegetables similar to pumpkin are carrots, broccoli, tomatoes, onions, and salad greens, which contain only a small amount of carbohydrate but are packed with micronutrients. They should be considered "free" foods for everyone. Eat them to your heart's content.

If additional fat and protein cause lower glycemic responses, shouldn't you advocate higher-protein or higher-fat diets for people with diabetes?

No, because *very* high-fat or high-protein diets have been associated with insulin resistance, which is obviously a problem for diabetics. This means that over the long term the consumption of any carbohydrate that accompanies fat or protein will tend to greatly increase blood glucose and insulin levels and cause deterioration in overall blood glucose control. More moderate increases in protein and fat (particularly **monounsaturated fat**) *may* be okay from a nutritional standpoint, but there hasn't been enough research conducted in order to say for sure.

Would someone with diabetes need to reduce their insulin dose if they changed to low-GI foods?

Most studies have not shown a need for a significantly reduced insulin dose when consuming a low-GI diet. This is probably because the insulin dose is dictated not just by carbohydrates in the diet but by protein and fat as well. A few initial studies of subjects using insulin pumps have suggested that they could reduce their insulin dosage and maintain the same blood glucose levels, but further research is needed to confirm this.

I have type 2 diabetes. How can I feed a big family with cost-effective, no-hassle, low-GI foods?

Feeding a big family on a budget can be hard. But low-GI eating often means making a move back to the inexpensive, filling, and healthy staple foods that your parents and grandparents may have enjoyed: traditional oats in oatmeal for breakfast; legumes such as beans, chickpeas, and lentils (all available dry or, for expediency, in cans); cereal grains like barley, and plenty of fresh fruits and vegetables, which have a naturally low GI.

Some of these foods may take a little more time to prepare than high-GI processed, packaged, and more expensive convenience foods, but you will save money and reap immeasurable health benefits, and many of these foods will keep you and your family firing with energy all day. In the GI tables in part 5, you'll find plenty of low-GI foods to choose from that won't break your budget. Your diabetes dietitian or educator will also have plenty of ideas for low-cost, low-GI meals that the whole family will enjoy.

I have diabetes, but I enjoy an occasional drink. Is that a problem?

First, see our answer above to the question, "What's the GI of alcoholic beverages?" (pages 157–158). Recent research has shown that a predinner drink tends to produce a "priming" effect, flicking the switch from internal to external sources of fuel and keeping blood sugar levels low. In one study, researchers gave healthy, young, lean people two standard glasses of beer, wine, a gin and tonic, or water to drink about an hour before eating a meal. Then their blood glucose and insulin levels were measured. The researchers found that "realistic amounts of beer, wine or gin reduce postmeal glucose levels, but not insulin levels."

■ Q&A's About GI, Blood Glucose, ■ and Other Metabolic Processes

I understand that low-GI foods help keep blood glucose low. What's wrong with high blood glucose levels?

High blood glucose levels pose a threat to your health. In fact, long before people may realize that their blood glucose levels are high, and before they are diagnosed with diabetes, moderately elevated blood glucose levels can damage the heart and circulatory system, increasing the risk of a heart attack, type 2 diabetes, weight gain, and even certain types of cancer.

Over time, the effects of high blood glucose levels become even more noticeable. Problems may occur with the skin, leading to bacterial infections, fungal infections, and itching. Nerves may be damaged, causing numbness, prickling, tingling, burning, and aching sensations. There may even be a loss of nerve function so that a process like digestion is impaired. The narrowing of large blood vessels will slow blood flow and cause heart disease, stroke, and the loss of circulation, which can lead to amputation. Small blood vessels may become damaged, which can cause problems that may include blurry vision, blindness, and kidney disease.

For all of these reasons, we advise eating a diet rich in low-GI foods, which, as we hope you now fully understand, helps to control blood glucose levels in people with and without diabetes, and can ward off both short- and long-term health problems.

What is the effect of extra protein and fat on blood glucose response?

Eaten alone, protein and fat have little effect on blood glucose levels. So a steak or a piece of cheese, for example, won't produce an increase in blood glucose. It's the *carbohydrate* in foods that is primarily responsible for the rise and fall in glucose after meals. Adding fat and protein to a meal doesn't affect the nature of the carbohydrate, and therefore does not affect its GI value.

But protein and fat will affect your blood glucose response when they're eaten along with carbohydrate. Both fat and protein tend to cause a delay in stomach emptying, thereby slowing the rate at which carbohydrate can be digested and absorbed. So a high-fat meal may have a lower glycemic effect—although not necessarily a different GI—than a low-fat meal, even if they both contain the same amount and type of carbohydrate.

Does low carb automatically mean low GI?

Not at all. Here's why: low carb is only about *quantity*; it simply means that a food or meal does not contain much carbohydrate. It says nothing about the *quality* of the carbs in the food or the meal on your plate. You could be eating a low-carb meal but the carbs could have a medium or high GI. Low GI, on the other hand, is all about quality.

Whether you are a moderate-carb or high-carb eater, low-GI carbs will have significant health benefits, as we detail throughout this book: promoting weight control, reducing your blood and insulin levels throughout the day, and increasing your sense of feeling full and satisfied after eating. We suggest that you make the most of quality carbs and reap the add-on health benefits, such as:

- vitamin E from whole-grain cereals
- vitamin C, beta-carotene, and potassium from fruits and vegetables
- vitamin B_6 from bananas and whole-grain cereals
- pantothenic acid, zinc, iron, and magnesium from whole grains and legumes
- antioxidants and phytochemicals from all plant foods
- fiber, which comes from all of the above and is not found in any animal food

If carbohydrates increase my blood glucose level, wouldn't a low-carbohydrate diet make sense?

The difficulty with this proposition is that there's hardly a shred of scientific evidence that a very low carb intake benefits anyone. In fact, as we mention throughout this book, there is strong evidence to suggest that moderate-to-high-carbohydrate diets are better for your health and easier to sustain.

Some popular diets are based on the concept of avoiding carbohydrate-based foods—even fruits and vegetables are restricted—

while meat and dairy foods laden with saturated fat, cholesterol, and calories form the basis of the diet. (Remember, a gram of fat has 9 calories, a gram of carbohydrate has 4.) This is a recipe for health problems; a wealth of research confirms that diets high in saturated fat are bad for your heart and can cause obesity.

Low-carb diets come in many forms, however. Some are not as extreme as that described above. The Zone diet, for example, recommends less carbohydrate (about 40 percent instead of 55 percent) and more protein (30 percent instead of 15 percent) but keeps fats to no more than 30 percent. It includes advice about quality of carbohydrate (low versus high GI) and type of fat (unsaturated versus saturated). To keep within the recommended limits, many specially prepared and packaged foods are often necessary. If you enjoy this way of eating, then there's nothing really wrong with it. But over time you may find yourself yearning for higher-carb foods like bread and potatoes.

One recent study from the Netherlands supported a diet with a moderate increase in protein (from 15 to 25 percent) and a moderate decrease in carbohydrate (from 55 to 45 percent). Fat intake was the same in both the control group and the high-protein group—30 percent of energy (calories). Volunteers in the study were allowed to eat as much food as they wished, but all were trying to lose weight. At the end of the twelve-week study, both weight loss and body-fat loss were greater in the high-protein group. The investigators suggested that the higher protein intake had increased the metabolic rate and also increased satiety. It is well known that protein stimulates more *thermogenesis* (heat production) than any other nutrient and is also the most satiating nutrient. There was no advice about the GI on either diet.

The glycemic index has been criticized because of variability in blood glucose responses between people and in the same person from day to day. How much variation should we expect? How much is okay?

When we measure the GI of a food in a group of individuals, not everyone produces the same GI. For example, if we test apples (average GI = 38), then one individual might give 20 and another 60. This is a natural biological variation that has been traced back to day-to-day variability in glucose tolerance, even in the same individual. One of the reasons we test the reference food three times in any one person is to obtain a reliable indication of their *normal* glucose tolerance. If we tested apples three times, we would also find that each person moved closer to the average result for the whole group. The bottom line is that foods classified as being high, medium, or low GI will show the same ranking in different individuals (as shown in figure 9).

This natural variability in blood glucose response has been a major source of criticism of the glycemic index. But it is illogical to criticize the glycemic index on these grounds, because the variability applies to *every* dietary approach, whether it be carbohydrate exchanges, carbohydrate counting, or a lower-carbohydrate diet. You can rely on the published GI value as a reliable ranking of foods, reflecting how you as an individual will respond to different foods most of the time.

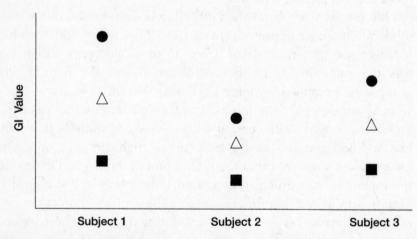

FIGURE 9. Three foods with high (●), intermediate (△), and low (■) GI values will follow the same ranking in different individuals.

Does it matter if you eat carbs after 5 PM?

Absolutely no scientific evidence supports the idea of not eating carbohydrates—or any foods, for that matter—after 5 PM, 8 PM, or any other time. People with diabetes who are taking insulin or other blood glucose–lowering medication, in particular, should *definitely* not practice a "carb curfew." If you want to reduce your total caloric intake, the better strategy, beyond eating fewer calories, is to eat low-GI carbohydrates, which will make you feel fuller longer and reduce hunger pangs.

I have recently been diagnosed with celiac disease (gluten sensitivity) on top of diabetes. It's extremely hard to find both low-GI and wheat-free foods. Any suggestions?

Good news: finding such foods may not be as hard as you think (or as it once was). Many Far East and Southeast Asian foods—Indian dals, stir-fries served with rice, sushi, and noodles—are all low GI. Vermicelli noodles prepared from rice or mung beans and low-GI rices, such as basmati, also meet your needs. Feel free to eat as many vegetables as you choose, while picking low-GI fruits. If you can eat dairy products without a problem, then take advantage of their universal low-GI values. On the other hand, if lactose intolerance is a problem, try yogurt with active cultures and lactose-free milk. Even ice cream can be enjoyed if you ingest a few drops of lactase enzyme (Lactaid) first. The GI tables in part 5 include a section on gluten-free foods (see page 304).

I've read that dairy products cause an increase in insulin secretion. Their GI is around 30–50, but their insulin index is three times higher.

Scientists don't know the reason that dairy products do this. Our guess is that milk proteins stimulate insulin secretion (they are said to be insulinogenic), because they are meant to stimulate the growth of young mammals. Insulin is a growth hormone designed to drive nutrients into cells—not just glucose but also fatty acids and amino acids, the building blocks of new tissue. Milk may contain a unique combination of amino acids that together are more insulin stimulating than any alone. This disparity between glucose and insulin response is not unique to dairy products. We've found that certain sweets and baked products also do this. Chocolate may also contain amino acids that stimulate insulin secretion.

How relevant is the GI for athletes?

"The glycemic index can be a useful tool to help athletes select the right type of carbohydrates to consume both before and after exercise," says Dr. Emma Stevenson. Several studies have investigated the effect on fuel usage during prolonged endurance exercise of changing the GI of carbohydrates eaten before exercise. Studies have consistently reported that a low-GI preexercise meal results in a better maintenance of blood glucose concentrations during exercise and a higher rate of fat burning. This is likely to reduce reliance on muscle carbohydrate stores during prolonged exercise and possibly improve endurance performance. Eating a high-GI meal before exercise may result in a glucose spike before the onset of exercise and then hypoglycemia occurring within the first thirty minutes of exercise. There is little information available on the effect of the GI of carbohydrates eaten before intermittent, power, or strength-related sports.

During recovery from exercise, replenishing muscle stores of carbohydrate is of high metabolic priority. Eating high-GI carbohydrates after exercise increases plasma glucose and insulin concentrations and this facilitates muscle glycogen resynthesis. If however, you are exercising for weight-loss purposes or are involved in weight-restricted sports, low-GI carbohydrates after exercise may be more beneficial because the lower glucose and insulin concentrations will not aid in fat burning.

■ Advanced Q&A's, ■
Especially for Clinicians and Other Researchers

Does the area under the curve give a true picture of the blood glucose response? What about the shape of the curve and the size of the glycemic spike?

The area under the curve (see "The GI Testing Protocol on page 10) may not be perfect, but it's thought to give the best summary measure of the overall degree of hyperglycemia experienced after eating. In research studies, the postprandial (post-meal) area under the curve has correlated strongly with measures such as glycated hemoglobin (HbA1c) that are related to risk of complications. In fact, recent studies have surprised even the experts, because the findings show that postprandial glycemia influences overall control much more than fasting or pre-meal blood glucose levels. Glycemic spikes appear to be important, too, but there is a close relation between the area under the curve and the peak response. If one is high, the other is high; conversely, if one is low, the other is low.

If testing were continued long enough, wouldn't you expect the areas under the curve to become equal, even for very high- and very low-GI foods?

Many people assume that if the amount of carbohydrate in two foods is the same, then the areas under the curve will ultimately be the same. This isn't the case, though, because the body is not only absorbing glucose from the gut into the bloodstream, but it is also *extracting* glucose from the blood. Just as a garden can utilize a gentle rain better than a sudden deluge, the body can metabolize slowly digested food better than quickly digested carbohydrate. Fast-release carbohydrate causes "flooding" of the system, and the body cannot extract the glucose from the blood fast enough. Just as water levels rise quickly after a torrential rain, so do glucose levels in the blood. But the same amount of rain falling over a longer period can be absorbed into the ground, and water levels do not rise.

Isn't the insulin response more important than the GI value? Wouldn't it be better to have an insulin index of foods rather than a glycemic index?

The insulin demand exerted by foods is indeed important for long-term health, but it doesn't necessarily follow that we need an insulin index of foods instead of a glycemic index. When they have been tested together, the glycemic index is extremely good at predicting a food's insulin index. (In other words, a low-GI food has a low insulin index value and a high-GI food has a high insulin index value.) There are some instances, however, in which a food has a low GI but a high insulin index value. This applies to dairy foods and to some highly palatable, energy-dense "indulgence foods." Some foods (such as meat, fish, and eggs) that contain no carbohydrate, just protein and fat (and have a GI of essentially zero), still stimulate significant increases in blood insulin.

We don't currently know how to interpret this type of response for long-term health. It may be a good outcome, because the increase in insulin has contributed to the low level of glycemia. On the other hand, it may be less than ideal, because the increased demand for insulin contributes to beta-cell "exhaustion" and the development of type 2 diabetes. Until studies are carried out to answer these types of questions, the glycemic index remains a proven dietary tool for predicting the effects of food on health.

Why are glucose and white bread used as test foods in GI testing— why not only glucose?

In the past, some scientists used a 50-gram carbohydrate portion of white bread as the reference food, because it was more typical of what we actually eat. On this scale, where the GI value of white bread is set at 100, some foods will have a GI value of over 100, because their effect on blood glucose levels is higher than that of bread.

The use of two standards has caused some confusion, so the glucose = 100 scale is now recommended. It is possible to convert from the bread scale to the glucose scale using the factor 0.7 (70 ÷ 100). This factor is derived from the fact that the GI value of white bread is 70 on the glucose = 100 scale.

To avoid confusion throughout this book, we refer to all foods according to a standard whereby glucose equals 100.

PART 4

Your Guide to Low-GI Eating

Simple tips to help you change to a low-GI diet, including a

how-to guide for vegetarians and more than 45 delicious

recipes to help you enjoy low-GI foods.

·14·

Making the Change to a Low-GI Diet

*L*ow-GI diets are easy to follow—a fact that may surprise you if you've struggled to adhere to other nutrition programs. That's because the basic technique is simple: replace high-GI foods in your diet with low-GI foods. This could mean eating oatmeal for breakfast instead of cornflakes, whole-grain bread instead of white, or fruit and/or yogurt in place of cookies, for example. But to make modifying the GI of your diet even easier, we've identified some other key points that are crucial in putting the GI into practice:

The glycemic index relates *only* to carbohydrate-rich foods.

The foods we eat contain three main macronutrients—protein, carbohydrate, and fat. Some foods, such as meat and eggs, are high in protein, while bread is high in carbohydrate, and butter is high in fat. It's important to consume a variety of foods, in varying proportions, to provide all three macronutrients—but the GI applies *only* to high-carbohydrate foods. (That's why we stress that the GI approach is only one element, and not the only criterion of a healthy diet.) As we've previously explained, it's impossible for us to measure the GI for foods that contain negligible amounts of carbohydrate, such as meat, fish, chicken, eggs, cheese, nuts, oils, cream, butter, and most vegetables. There are other nutritional aspects to consider when choosing these foods, though. For example, the amount and type of fats they have is significant, as is the amount of calories they contain.

The glycemic index is not intended to be used in isolation.

A food's GI does not make it "good" or "bad." High-GI foods, such as potatoes and bread, still make a valuable nutritional contribution to your diet. Plus, there are many low-GI foods, such as sausage, that are high in saturated fat and therefore not particularly healthful. The nutritional benefits of different foods are many and varied, and it is advisable for you to base your food choices on the overall nutritional content of a food, taking into consideration the saturated fat, salt, fiber, calorie content, and GI.

There's no need to eat only low-GI foods.

While most of us will benefit from eating low-GI carbs at each meal, this doesn't mean we need to consume them at the exclusion of all other carbs. When we eat a combination of high- and low-GI carbs—like cornflakes and strawberries, rice and beans, or potatoes and corn—the final GI of the meal is intermediate, or medium. That's because the high-GI value of foods such as potato is moderated by including a low-GI carb at the same meal. For example, if your main meal contains a baked potato (GI = 77), then choose a low-GI dessert, such as low-fat yogurt with no added sugar (GI = 20). Let's assume that half the carbohydrate comes from the potato and half from the yogurt. The GI value for the meal then becomes (50% $\times$ 77) + (50% $\times$ 20) = 49.

Consider both a food's GI and the amount of carbohydrate it contains (i.e., its glycemic load).

For some foods, the normal serving size contains so little carbohydrate that its GI is insignificant. This is generally the case for vegetables like carrots (41), green peas (48), and pumpkin (75), which provide about 6 grams of carbohydrate per serving. Small amounts of jam (46–50) or commercial-blend honey (64) also have little glycemic impact. You can calculate a food's GL by multiplying its GI by the amount of carbohydrate in that particular food for a particular serving size and then dividing by 100. (See "Glycemic Index or Glycemic Load?" on page 16 for a fuller discussion of GL.). We've also included the GL of foods in the GI tables in part 5; you can browse through the table to see how a food's GL differs from its GI.

■ The 7 Guidelines of Low-GI Eating ■

Choosing low-GI foods is one of *the* most important dietary choices you can make. As well as identifying your best low-GI, smart-carb choices, our seven dietary guidelines below give you a blueprint for eating for life.

> **1.** Eat seven or more servings of fruits and vegetables every day.
> **2.** Eat low-GI breads and cereals.
> **3.** Eat more legumes, including soybeans, chickpeas, and lentils.
> **4.** Eat nuts more regularly.
> **5.** Eat more fish and seafood.
> **6.** Eat lean red meats, poultry, and eggs.
> **7.** Eat low-fat dairy products.

1. Eat seven or more servings of fruits and vegetables every day.

Why? Being high in fiber, and therefore filling, and low in fat (apart from olives and avocado, which contain some "good" fats), fruits and vegetables play a central role in eating the low-GI way. In addition to protecting you against diseases (ranging from high blood pressure to cancer), they are bursting with nutrients that will give you a glow of good health, such as:

Beta-carotene—the plant precursor of vitamin A, which is used to maintain healthy skin and eyes. A diet rich in beta-carotene may even lessen skin damage caused by UV rays. Apricots, peaches, mangoes, carrots, broccoli, and sweet potatoes are particularly rich in beta-carotene.

Vitamin C—nature's water-soluble antioxidant. Antioxidants are a little like your personal bodyguard, protecting your body cells from the damage that can be caused by pollutants in our environment and that also occurs as a natural part of aging. Guava, peppers, orange, kiwi fruit, and cantaloupe are especially rich in vitamin C.

Anthocyanins—the purple and red pigments in blueberries, peppers, beets, and eggplant that also function as antioxidants, minimizing the damage to cell membranes that occurs with aging.

How much? Aim to eat at least two servings of fruit and five servings of vegetables every day, preferably of three or more different colors. A serving is about one medium-sized piece of fruit, half a cup of cooked vegetables, or 1 cup of raw veggies.

Which vegetables are low GI? Most vegetables contain so little carbohydrate that they don't have a GI value. Potato is a notable exception, however—it has a high GI. If you are a big potato eater, try to replace some of the potato in your diet with these low-GI alternatives.

Sweet corn (GI = 46–48). Sweet corn contains folic acid, potassium, the antioxidant vitamins A and C, and dietary fiber. Add canned or frozen kernels to soups, stews, relishes, salsas, and salads, or simply enjoy it on the cob. For the best flavor, buy fresh corn with the husk intact, because the sugar in the kernels is transformed into starch the moment the husk is removed.

Corn is often used as a base for gluten-free products. However, many products manufactured from corn, such as cornflakes, cornmeal, and corn pasta, do not have a low GI. Check the GI table first.

Sweet potato (GI = 46). An excellent source of beta-carotene, vitamin C, and dietary fiber, sweet potatoes make a great substitute for potatoes. Peel them or simply scrub the skins and steam, boil, bake, or microwave. Try mashing them with a little mustard seed oil or wrapping them in foil and cooking on the grill. They also make a tasty addition to casseroles, stir-fries, and soups, and (roasted first) to salads.

Taro (GI = 54). A traditional, slowly digested food eaten widely throughout the Pacific Islands, taro has a dry texture, a flavor similar to sweet potato, and can be used the same way. Before cooking, peel off the thick skin (wearing rubber gloves, as the juice has been known to cause skin irritation), then cut into wedges and steam, boil, or bake.

Yam (GI = 37). Sold in North America mostly in specialty Asian and Caribbean grocers, yams are similar to sweet potato and taro but have an earthier flavor. High in fiber and nutrient dense, yams can be steamed, microwaved, boiled, or baked in wedges, or roasted and added to salads.

Fruit. Most fruits have a low GI, thanks to the presence of the low-GI sugar fructose, soluble and insoluble fibers, and acids (which may slow down stomach emptying). The lowest-GI fruits—apples, pears, all citrus (oranges, grapefruit, mandarins) and stone fruits (peaches, nectarines, plums, apricots)—are those grown in temperate climates. Generally, the more acidic a fruit, the lower the GI.

Tropical fruits, such as pineapple, cantaloupe, and watermelon, tend to have intermediate GI values, but they are excellent sources of antioxidants, and in average servings their GL is low.

Most berries have so little carbohydrate that their GI is impossible to test. Strawberries have been tested, however, and they are low GI. Enjoy them by the bowl.

2. Eat low-gi breads and cereals.

Why? What affects the GI of your diet the most? The type of bread and cereals you eat. Mixed-grain breads, sourdough, traditional rolled oats, cracked wheat, pearl barley, pasta, noodles, and certain types of rice are just some examples of low-GI cereal foods. The slow digestion and absorption of these foods will fill you up more, trickle fuel into your engine at a more useable rate, and keep you satisfied for longer.

How much? Most people need at least five servings of grains each day (very active people need much more); a serving is one slice of bread or ½ cup of cooked rice, pasta, or noodles.

Bread. Bread forms an important part of most people's diets. One of the most important changes you can make to lower the GI of your diet is to choose a low-GI bread. Choose a really grainy bread, stone-ground or whole-grain bread, sourdough bread, or bread made from chickpea or other legume-based flours. Small, artisanal bakeries are the most likely places you will find them. Some healthy, low-GI choices are listed below.

Whole-grain breads. Whole-grain breads contain lots of grainy pieces, tend to be chewy, and are nutritionally superior, containing high levels of fiber, vitamins, minerals, and phytoestrogens.

Choose breads made with whole cereal grains such as barley, rye, triticale (a hybrid of wheat and rye), oats, soy, and cracked wheat, and have seeds such as sunflower, sesame, or flax added.

Pumpernickel. Also known as rye kernel bread, pumpernickel contains 80 to 90 percent whole and cracked rye kernels. It is dense and compact and is usually sold thinly sliced. The main reason for its low GI value is its content of whole cereal grains.

Sourdough. Sourdough results from the deliberately slow fermentation of flour by yeasts, which produces a buildup of organic acids. These acids give sourdough its characteristic taste. This flavorful low-GI bread is a popular choice for sandwiches (its compact structure keeps the sandwich intact), makes great toast, and is generally considered acceptable by those family members who absolutely insist on white bread. The flavor blends well with all kinds of fillings and toppings, making it ideal for lunch boxes, snacks, and to serve with soups, salads, and main meals.

Stone-ground or whole-wheat breads. This means that the flour has been milled from the entire wheat berry (the germ, endosperm or starch compartment, and the bran) and that the milling process uses a method of slowly grinding the grain with a burr stone instead of high-speed metal rollers to distribute the germ oil more evenly. Virtually none of the ingredients packaged in the wheat berry get lost in this processing method, and that is why this bread is such a rich source of several B vitamins, iron, zinc, and dietary fiber.

Fruit bread. The GI of fruit bread is relatively low because of the part substitution of wheat flour (high GI) with dried fruits (lower GI). The presence of sugar in the dough also limits gelatinization of the starch.

Chapatti-baisen. Chapatti is unleavened or slightly leavened bread that looks rather like pita bread. It is widely eaten throughout the Indian subcontinent and is available in Indian restaurants world-wide. While it is often made with wheat flour, it is also made from baisen or chickpea flour, giving it a significantly lower GI (27) than that made from wheat flour (63), due to the nature of the starch. All legumes, including chickpeas, have a higher proportion of amylose starch than that found in cereal grains. So before you order, ask what kind of flour was used.

Breakfast cereals. Traditional rolled oats cooked into oatmeal is about the closest most of us come to a true whole-grain cereal. Although many commercial cereals are labeled "whole-grain," the processing they have undergone has destroyed the original physical form of the grain. Some commercial breakfast cereals, however, still do have a low GI, thanks to a less extreme degree of processing and the presence of other factors (such as protein or soluble fiber) that slow down digestion. Or try making your own muesli using rolled oats and a mixture of dried fruit, nuts, and seeds.

Other Low-GI Cereal Grains

Barley (GI = 25). One of the oldest cultivated cereals, barley is very nutritious and high in soluble fiber, which helps to reduce the post-meal rise in blood glucose and lowers its GI. Look for products such as pearl barley to use in soups, stews, and pilafs, and barley flakes or rolled barley, which have a light, nutty flavor and can be cooked as a cereal and used in baked goods and stuffing.

Bulgur (GI = 48). Also known as cracked wheat, bulgur is made from wheat grains that have been hulled and steamed before grinding to crack the grain. The whole-wheat grain in bulgur remains virtually intact—it is simply cracked—and the wheat germ and bran are retained, which preserves nutrients and lowers the GI. Bulgur is used as the base of the Middle Eastern salad tabbouleh, but can also be used in pilafs, veggie burgers, stuffing, stews, salads, and soups, or as a cereal.

Noodles. Many Asian noodles, such as Hokkien, udon, and rice vermicelli, have a low to intermediate GI because of their dense texture, whether they are made from wheat or rice flour. Lungkow bean thread noodles (GI = 35), also called cellophane noodles or green bean vermicelli, are a smart carb choice. These shiny, fine, white noodles are usually sold in bundles wrapped in cellophane in the Asian food aisle of your supermarket or in an Asian food market. Soak them in hot water for ten minutes, then add to a stir-fry or salad, as they tend to absorb the flavors of other foods they are cooked with. They have a low GI thanks to their legume origin (they're made from mung beans) and their noodle shape and dense texture.

Oats (GI = 58). Rolled oats are whole-grain oats that have been hulled, steamed, and flattened; this popular cereal grain lowers the GI of oatmeal, muesli, cookies, bread, and meatloaf. Oat bran also has a low GI.

Pasta. Pastas of any shape or size have a fairly low GI and are a great standby for quick meals. Served with vegetables or tomato sauce and/or accompaniments, such as olive oil, fish, and lean meat, plenty of vegetables, and small amounts of cheese, a pasta meal gives you a healthy balance of carbs, fats, and proteins. Pasta should be slightly firm (al dente) and offer some resistance when you are chewing it.

Not only does it taste better this way, but it also has a lower GI, which overcooking boosts. While pasta is a good low-GI choice, a huge amount will have a marked effect on your blood glucose. Remember, a standard portion of cooked pasta is one cup, which may be less than what you are used to eating.

Most pasta is made from semolina (finely cracked wheat), which is milled from very hard wheat (durum) with a high protein content. There is some evidence that thicker types of pasta have a lower GI than thinner types because of the dense consistency, and perhaps because they cook more slowly and are less likely to be overcooked. Adding egg to fresh pasta lowers the GI by increasing the protein content.

Note: Canned spaghetti has a higher GI value than other types of pasta.

Rice. Rice can have a high GI value (80–109) or a low GI value (50–55), depending on the variety and, in particular, its amylose content.

Basmati rice (GI = 58) and Uncle Ben's converted, long-grain rice (GI = 50), and Uncle Ben's long grain and wild rice blend (GI = 57) contain higher proportions of amylose (a type of starch that we digest more slowly), which produces a lower glycemic response, is more compact in structure and more slowly digested.

Arborio rice, which is especially good for making Italian risotto, releases its starch during cooking and, as a result, has a higher GI. Waxy or glutinous rice, often used for rice desserts as it becomes sticky when cooked, has a high GI. Eat less of these kinds of rice.

> **Sushi (GI = 48)**—These bite-size parcels of raw or smoked fish, chicken, tofu, and/or pickled, raw, or cooked vegetables wrapped in seaweed with rice that has been seasoned with vinegar, salt, and sugar make ideal snacks and light meals. Even though the rice that is used to make sushi can sometimes be short grain and somewhat sticky, sushi is low GI. In addition, sushi made with salmon and tuna boosts your intake of the healthy omega-3 fats.

Rye (GI = 34). Whole-kernel rye is used to make certain breads, including pumpernickel and some crispbreads. Rye flakes can be used in a similar way to rolled oats: you can eat them as a cooked cereal or sprinkle them over bread before you bake it.

Whole wheat kernels (GI = 41). Wheat is a staple food to half the world's population. Soak whole wheat overnight and simmer for about an hour to use as a base for pilaf. Some people enjoy wheat bran as a cooked breakfast cereal. Cream of wheat is made from very fine semolina; you can use it as a breakfast cereal or in puddings, custards, soufflés, and soups.

3. Eat more legumes, including soybeans, chickpeas, and lentils.

Why? Look no further than legumes for a low-GI food that is easy on the budget, versatile, filling, nutritious, and low in calories. Legumes are high in fiber, too—both soluble and insoluble—and are packed with nutrients, providing a valuable source of protein, carbohydrate, B vitamins, iron, zinc, and magnesium. Whether you buy dried beans, lentils, and chickpeas and cook them yourself at home, or opt for the very convenient, time-saving canned varieties, you are choosing one of nature's lowest-GI foods.

Legumes have two particularly special properties in their armory of health benefits. The first is their content of phytochemicals, natural plant chemicals that possess antiviral, antifungal, antibacterial, and anticancer properties. Second, legumes are prebiotics. This means that they provide food for our gut bacteria, or "intestinal flora," keeping our digestive systems healthy.

A bean meal doesn't always have to be strictly vegetarian. Try using beans in place of grains or potatoes. You can serve a bean salsa with fish or cannellini bean purée with grilled meat. Butter beans can also make a delicious potato substitute. Although they will keep indefinitely, it is best to use dried legumes within one year of purchase.

How much? At least twice a week as a main meal, such as bean soup, chickpea curry, or lentil patties, or as a light meal, such as beans on toast, mixed-bean salad, or pea and ham soup.

Beans. When you add beans to meals and snacks, you reduce the overall GI of your diet and gain important health benefits. Beans are available dried or in cans. Young beans cook faster than old ones and will also be more vividly colored. Substitute one 14-ounce can of beans for three-quarters of a cup of dried beans. Dried beans usually have a lower GI than canned, but using canned beans is much more convenient and the GI remains low.

Baked beans	GI = 49
Black-eyed peas	GI = 42
Butter beans (dried, boiled, not canned)	GI = 31
Cannellini beans	GI = 31
Haricot beans	GI = 33
Lima beans	GI = 32
Mung beans	GI = 39
Red kidney beans	GI = 36

Chickpeas (dried, boiled, not canned) (GI = 28). Popular in Middle Eastern and Mediterranean dishes, these large, caramel-colored legumes are available in cans or as dried beans. To cook chickpeas, first place them in a bowl, cover them with plenty of cold water, and soak them overnight. Drain the water, then put the chickpeas in a saucepan and cover them with clean water. Bring the beans to a boil for ten minutes, then simmer for 1½ hours until they're tender to bite.

You can also roast and salt whole chickpeas for a delicious snack food. (Wasabi chickpeas are now widely available in specialty and health-oriented food markets.) Ground chickpea flour, also called baisen, is used to make unleavened Indian bread.

Lentils (GI = 26–48). Rich in protein, fiber, and B vitamins, all colors and types of lentils have a similarly low GI, which is increased slightly if you buy them canned and add them at the end of cooking time. Lentils are one food that people with diabetes should learn to love— they can eat them until the cows come home. In fact, we have found that no matter how much of them people eat, they have only a small effect on blood glucose levels. Lentils have a fairly bland, earthy flavor and are best prepared with onions, garlic, and spices. Use them as a "bed" for grilled fish or meat. They are great for thickening any kind of soup or extending meat casseroles.

Channa dal (also called Bengal gram dal) are husked, split, polished beans (GI = 11), the most common type of gram lentil in India. They are often cooked with a pinch of asafetida (an Indian spice) to make them easier to digest.

Dried Legume Preparation

1. **Soak.** Place legumes in a saucepan and cover them with two to three times their volume of cold water. Soak them overnight or during the day.

   Shortcut: Rather than soaking overnight, add three times the volume of water to rinsed beans, bring to a boil for a few minutes, then remove from heat and let soak for an hour. Drain, add fresh water, then cook as usual.

2. **Cook.** Drain off the soaking water, adding two to three times the volume of water as beans. Bring the water to a boil, then simmer until beans are tender. Use the directions on the packet or the information below as a time guide.

   - Don't add salt to the cooking water—it slows down water absorption so cooking takes longer.
   - Don't cook beans in the water they have soaked in. Substances that contribute to flatulence are leached from the beans into the soaking and cooking waters.

   Shortcuts: Precooked canned legumes make cooking with beans quick and easy. Legume-based meals come together much faster than those based on meat.

Precook your own dried legumes and freeze them in small batches. You can keep soaked or cooked beans in an airtight container for several days in the fridge.

Soybeans (canned, drained) (GI = 14). An excellent source of protein, soybeans and soy products have been a staple part of Asian diets for thousands of years. They're also rich in fiber, iron, zinc, and vitamin B, and they're lower in carbohydrate and higher in fat than other legumes, although the majority of the fat is polyunsaturated. Soy is also a rich source of phytochemicals—phytoestrogens in particular—which are plant estrogens with a structure similar to the female hormone estrogen. Some studies link phytoestrogens with improvements in blood cholesterol levels, relief from menopausal symptoms, and lower rates of cancer.

Split peas (GI = 32). Prepared from a variety of the common garden pea with the husk removed, split peas may be yellow or green. They take about an hour or so to cook after soaking (depending on their age) and are traditionally used in pea and ham soups or for making an Indian dal.

4. Eat nuts more regularly.

Why? Although nuts are high in fat, it is mainly polyunsaturated and monounsaturated, so they make a healthy substitute for less nutritious, snacks that are high in saturated fat, such as potato chips, chocolate, and cookies.

Nuts are one of the richest sources of vitamin E, which, with the selenium they contain, works as an antioxidant. Selenium helps guard against harmful UV rays to reduce both damage caused by the sun and premature aging of your skin.

How much? Aim for a small handful of nuts (1 ounce) most days. Here are some easy ways to eat more nuts:

▶ Use nuts and seeds in food preparation. For example, use toasted cashews or sesame seeds in a chicken stir-fry; sprinkle walnuts or pine nuts over a salad; top fruity desserts or granola with almonds.

▶ Use hazelnut spread on bread or try peanut, almond, or cashew butter rather than butter or margarine.

▶ Sprinkle a mixture of ground nuts and flaxseeds over cereal or salads, or add to baked goods, such as muffins.

5. Eat more fish and seafood.

Why? Fish does not have a GI, as it is a source of protein and good fat, not carbohydrate. Increased fish consumption is linked to a reduced risk of coronary heart disease, improvements in mood, lower rates of depression, better blood-fat levels, and enhanced immunity. Just one serving of fish a week may reduce the risk of a fatal heart attack by 40 percent. The likely protective components of fish are the very-long-chain omega-3 fatty acids. Our bodies make only small amounts of these fatty acids, so we rely on dietary sources, especially fish and seafood, for them.

How much? One to three meals of fish each week.

Which fish is best?

- Oily fish, which tend to have darker-colored flesh and a stronger flavor, are the richest source of omega-3 fats.
- Canned salmon, sardines, mackerel, and, to a lesser extent, tuna are all very rich sources of omega-3's; look for canned fish packed in water, canola oil, olive oil, tomato sauce, or brine, and drain well.
- Fresh fish with higher levels of omega-3's are: Pacific and Atlantic salmon and smoked salmon; Atlantic and Pacific mackerel; and bluefin tuna. Eastern and Pacific oysters and squid (calamari) are also rich sources.

Mercury in Fish

DUE TO THE risk of high levels of mercury in certain species of fish, the Food and Drug Administration (FDA) has advised that pregnant women, nursing mothers, women planning pregnancy, and young children should avoid consuming certain species but can continue to consume a variety of fish as part of a healthy diet. Shark, swordfish, king mackerel, and tilefish should not be consumed, because these long-lived, larger fish contain the highest levels of mercury. Pregnant women should select a variety of other kinds of fish—shellfish, canned fish such as light tuna, smaller ocean fish, or farm-raised fish. The FDA recommends two 3 ounce servings per week, but that you can safely eat up to 12 ounces of cooked fish per week.

6. Eat lean red meats, poultry, and eggs.

Why? Again, these foods do not have a GI, because they are a protein food, not a carbohydrate. Red meat is the best source of iron (the nutrient used for carrying oxygen in our blood) you can get.

Good iron status can increase energy levels and improve our exercise tolerance. While adequate iron can be obtained from a vegetarian diet, women particularly must select foods carefully to prevent iron deficiency. A chronic shortage of iron leads to anemia, the symptoms of which include pale skin, excessive tiredness, breathlessness, irritability, and decreased attention span.

How much? We suggest eating lean meat two or three times a week, and accompanying it with a salad or vegetables. Three and one-half ounces of lean edible meat as part of a balanced diet will meet the daily nutrient needs of an adult, but larger amounts can also be part of a healthy diet. A couple of eggs or 4 ounces of skinless chicken provide options for variety once or twice a week.

7. Eat low-fat dairy products.

Why? Milk, cheese, ice cream, yogurt, buttermilk, pudding, and custard are the richest sources of calcium in our diet. Calcium is vital in many body functions, so if we don't get enough in our diet, the body will draw it out of our bones. This bone loss over a number of years may lead to osteoporosis and loss of height, curvature of the spine, and peridontal disease (deterioration of bones supporting the teeth). By replacing full-fat dairy foods with reduced-fat, low-fat, or fat-free versions, you will reduce your saturated fat intake and actually boost your calcium intake. Also, recent research shows that calcium and other components in dairy play a vital role in fat burning.

How much? To meet calcium requirements, experts recommend that adults eat two to three servings of dairy products every day. Good low-fat dairy choices include skim, fat-free, or low-fat milk and fat-free or low-fat yogurt. A serving is a cup of milk, 1 ounce of cheese, or 6 ounces of yogurt.

If you're lactose intolerant, you can still eat yogurt and cheese. You can also try lactose-reduced or lactose-free milk, high-calcium soy milk, salmon, high-calcium tofu, calcium-fortified breakfast cereal, and fresh or dried figs—all great-tasting nondairy sources of calcium.

A Sensible Approach to Shifting to a Low-GI Diet

UNLIKE GIVING UP bad habits, such as smoking, changing our diet is seldom just a matter of forgoing certain foods. Follow these four guidelines as you're making the change to a low-GI diet:

1. **Aim to make changes gradually.** Major changes to diet are usually short-lived—which is why few people can follow fad diets for long. Instead, identify one aspect of your diet that you want to work on (for example, eating more vegetables) and make that your focus. Once you've made the change and feel comfortable with it, then attempt to make the next adjustment in your diet, and so on.

2. **Attempt the easiest changes first.** Nothing inspires like success, so increase your chances by attacking the easiest changes first. For example, plan to eat one fruit snack each day, then move on to extra servings of vegetables, etc.

3. **Break down big goals into a number of smaller, more achievable goals.** A big goal may be wanting to lose a lot of weight. This is unlikely to happen quickly, but it is attainable through gradual, consistent change. Smaller goals could be to exercise for thirty minutes every day and to reduce the saturated-fat content of your diet. Even smaller goals (which are the way to begin) could be to do a fifteen-minute walk twice a week and limit takeout to once a week.

4. **Accept lapses in your habits.** Lapses are not failures but rather the natural stages in the progression to new habits. Remember, it usually takes about three months for a new change to become a habit.

Milk (GI = 12–14). Milk is a rich source of protein and vitamin B_2 (riboflavin). As whole milk is also a rich source of saturated fat, choose low-fat and fat-free milk and milk products. The surprisingly low GI of milk is a combination of the moderate GI effect of the lactose (milk sugar) plus the effect of the milk protein, which forms a soft curd in the stomach and slows down the rate of stomach emptying.

Yogurt (GI = 20–40). Yogurt is rich in calcium, riboflavin, and protein. Low-fat natural yogurt provides the most calcium for the fewest calories. The combination of yogurt's acidity and high protein contributes to its low GI. Fruit yogurts made with a sugar-sweetened fruit syrup have a GI of around 33, whereas artificially sweetened yogurts have a GI of around 14.

Low-fat ice cream (GI = 37–49). Low-fat ice cream is a delicious source of all the goodies found in milk. It is important that you choose a low-fat (< 3 grams of fat per 100 grams) variety for regular consumption so that you don't overdo your saturated fat intake. Save the gourmet varieties for an occasional indulgence. Ice cream has a slightly higher GI than milk because of the presence of sucrose and glucose in addition to lactose.

■ Putting the GI to Work During Your Day ■

Breakfast—sustaining you through the day

Research makes clear that people who eat breakfast are calmer, happier, and more effective at work—and that eating breakfast improves mood, mental alertness, concentration, and memory. It can also help people lose weight and lower their cholesterol levels, too. We also know it helps stabilize blood glucose levels.

By the same token, missing breakfast can cause fatigue, dehydration, and a loss of energy. Eating a high-GI breakfast is not the answer, though, as it can leave you hungry by mid-morning. Many breakfast cereals and breads are high GI, which means while they pick you up initially, the effect doesn't last long. When the energy runs out and your blood glucose starts to drop, you feel hungry again. By switching to low-GI breakfast choices, you'll see how much easier it is to make it through to lunchtime.

Three-quarters of people who skip breakfast say they have "no time to eat," so we include lots of quick, healthy, low-GI breakfast ideas. Whether you prefer a liquid breakfast on the go, a hearty hot breakfast, or simply a low-fat granola bar and an apple on the way to work, we guarantee you'll find something to sustain you through the day.

■

Skipping breakfast is not a good way to cut back on calories! Studies show that breakfast-skippers tend to make up for the missed food by eating more snacks during the day and more food overall.

■

■ Low-GI Breakfast Basics

1. Start with some fruit or juice.

Fruit contributes fiber and, more important, vitamin C, which helps your body absorb the nutrient iron.

LOWEST-GI FRESH FRUITS AND JUICES

Apples	38
Kiwi fruit	53
Apple juice	37–44
Mango	51
Banana	52
Orange	42
Carrot juice	43
Peach	42
Pear	38
Grapefruit	25
Pineapple juice	46
Grapefruit juice	48
Plum	39
Grapes	53
Tomato juice	38

2. Try a low-GI breakfast cereal.

Cereals are important as a source of fiber and vitamin B. When choosing processed breakfast cereals, look for those with a high fiber content. Scan the breakfast cereals entries in the GI tables in part 5 (on page 297).

3. Add milk or yogurt.

Low-fat milk or yogurt will make a valuable contribution to your daily calcium intake, and both have a low GI value. Lower-fat varieties have just as much, or more, calcium as regular types.

4. Add bread or toast if you are still hungry.

Choose truly whole-grain breads, made with intact kernels—see page 296 of the GI tables for low-GI breads.

■ Ten Delicious Low-GI Breakfasts ■

1. Toast a slice of pumpernickel, spread lightly with margarine and accompany with a hot chocolate drink made with low-fat milk.
2. Lightly toast some sourdough English muffins. Spread with natural peanut butter and spreadable fruit jam.
3. Add unsweetened canned peaches or applesauce to creamy oatmeal (made with fat-free or low-fat milk), sprinkle with cinnamon, and drizzle with a teaspoon of honey.
4. Pan-fry or toast a ham and part-skim melted cheese sandwich made with 100 percent stone-ground whole-wheat bread.
5. Top a bowl of vanilla-flavored, low-fat yogurt with a sliced peach and chopped strawberries, then scatter low-fat granola over the top.
6. Combine a 6-ounce container of low-fat fruit yogurt with 2 tablespoons of chopped almonds, 1 diced banana or pear, and 1 cup of Bran Buds. Serves two.
7. Spread a generous layer of Nutella or natural peanut butter on Ryvita¨ dark rye whole-grain crackers, and team it with a mug of low-fat caffè latte.

8. Beat together 2 eggs, ¼ cup of skim milk, and a teaspoon of pure vanilla extract. Dip 4 thick slices of sourdough bread into the egg mixture, then cook over medium heat in a greased, nonstick frying pan for 2 to 3 minutes each side, until golden. Serve topped with pan-fried pear or apple slices and a sprinkling of cinnamon.

9. Toast pita bread and top with fresh light ricotta and a dollop of blackberry all-fruit preserves.

10. Make a big bowl of steaming oatmeal, then stir in some frozen blueberries or raspberries. Top with a dollop of low-fat natural yogurt and a sprinkling of brown sugar.

■ Refueling with a Low-GI Lunch ■

It's important to refuel in the afternoon to keep your blood glucose—and your energy levels—even. Lunch needn't be a big meal, though. In fact, if you find yourself feeling sleepy after lunch, it may help to eat a lighter meal of protein, vegetables, and a small portion of carbohydrate. (A cup of coffee helps, too!)

Buying Lunch and Looking for a Low-GI Choice?

LOOK FOR ANY of the following low-GI lunch options. Many of the traditional dishes on ethnic-restaurant menus will have a low GI, because they are based on legumes.

- Sushi
- Moroccan couscous (with chickpeas)
- Rice noodle soup
- Tortilla with beans and tomato sauce
- Thai noodles with vegetables
- Lentil soup
- Stuffed grape leaves
- Ravioli
- Tabbouleh
- Lentils and rice
- Hummus

■ Low-GI Lunch Basics ■

▶ Carbohydrate-rich foods with a low GI value, such as whole-grain bread, pasta or noodles, grains or legumes.
▶ Proteins like fish, lean meat, chicken, cheese, or egg.
▶ Vegetables to bulk it out and fill you up. A large salad with a variety of vegetables would be ideal.
▶ Round it off with fruit.

■ Ten Light and Lively ■ Low-GI Lunch Ideas

You may think some of these recipes are too time-consuming, but if you want to improve the wholesomeness of your lunches and feel your best throughout the afternoon, these great ideas are worth the few minutes they'll take to prepare. Make extra for multiple servings.

1. Take a piece of pita bread, spread it with hummus, top with thinly sliced lean roast beef and tabbouleh, and roll up.
2. Make a lentil and sweet potato soup by browning an onion with 2 cloves of crushed garlic. Add 1 lb. sweet potato chunks, ½ cup of split red lentils, and 3½ cups of vegetable stock. Simmer for 25 minutes, adding 1 coarsely grated zucchini after 20 minutes.
3. Slice a sweet potato into very thin slices. Cut a zucchini in half lengthwise and cut a red onion into 6 segments. Place vegetables in a freezer bag with a clove of crushed garlic, add a tablespoon of olive oil, and shake to coat. Spread out on a baking sheet and roast in a hot oven 20–30 minutes until tender. Toss the roasted vegetables with boiled pasta, along with chopped parsley, oregano, or basil, and a drizzle of olive oil.
4. Divide a small package (8 oz) of tortilla chips (preferably a salt-reduced, low-fat variety from the health food section) among four ovenproof plates. Top with a 16-ounce can of Mexican or chili-flavored kidney beans and sprinkle with reduced-fat cheddar or Monterey Jack cheese. Put under a hot grill for 2–3 minutes, then top with dollops of mashed avocado.

5. Take a small (3 oz) can of tuna in spring water and ¼ cup of drained cannellini beans. Mix in a bowl with half a diced cucumber, 1 diced tomato, a handful of baby spinach (or other greens), and chopped parsley. Dress with an equal mix of olive oil and lemon juice and a sprinkling of black pepper.

6. Spread 1 slice of 100 percent whole-wheat bread with whole-grain mustard. Add chopped sundried tomatoes, grilled eggplant, and a slice of mozzarella cheese. Melt the cheese under a grill, then add salad greens and another slice of bread. Cut in half and serve.

7. Try canned salmon, thinly sliced green apple, and red onion with snow-pea sprouts on sourdough bread.

8. Sauté 2 sliced green onions with a teaspoon each of crushed garlic and ginger until soft (do not brown). Add 2–3 sliced mushrooms, 1 teaspoon of minced jalapeño, 1 tablespoon of soy sauce, and 1 teaspoon sesame oil and cook until the mushrooms soften. Add 1 cup of vegetable stock, bring to a boil, then stir in a package of Japanese noodles, diced cooked chicken or tofu, and a handful of shredded spinach.

9. Cook a half cup of split red lentils in boiling water until tender (about 10 minutes). Drain. When cool, mash with 2 tablespoons mayonnaise, 2 chopped green onions, and a clove of crushed garlic. Season with black pepper. Use on your favorite bread as a sandwich filling with salad greens.

10. Make a vegetarian chickpea burger by combining a can of drained chickpeas with fresh whole-wheat bread crumbs, parsley, garlic, and an egg in a food processor. Shape into patties and pan fry. Serve with char-grilled vegetables on a whole-wheat bun. You can also select from the fresh and frozen veggie burgers in your supermarket.

■ Low-GI Main Meals: ■
Choosing the Best

1, 2, 3 . . . Putting it on the plate

Main meals for most Americans consist of some sort of meat (or chicken or fish) with vegetables and potato (or rice or pasta). This is a good start, and a little fine-tuning will ensure a healthy, balanced meal. All you need to do is adjust your proportions to match our "plate." Here are the three simple steps to put together a balanced low-GI meal:

1 is for carb

It's an essential, although sometimes forgotten, part of a balanced meal. What do you feel like eating? A grain like rice, barley, or cracked wheat? Pasta, noodles, or whole-wheat spaghetti? Or perhaps a high-carb vegetable like sweet corn, sweet potato, or legumes?

Include at least one low-GI carb per meal.

2 is for protein

Include some protein at each meal. It lowers the glycemic load by replacing *some* of the carbohydrate—not all! It also helps satisfy the appetite.

3 is for fruits and vegetables

This is the part we often go without. If anything, it should have the highest priority in a meal, but a meal based solely on fruit and low-carb vegetables won't be sustaining for long. A plain salad is a recipe for hunger.

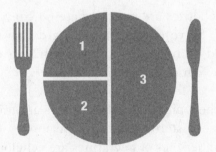
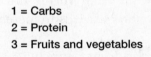

1 = Carbs
2 = Protein
3 = Fruits and vegetables

The plate model is adaptable to any serving sizes.

- As long you keep food to the proportions shown here, the meal will be balanced.
- As long as the types of food you choose fit within the guidelines for healthy eating, then you should have a healthy diet overall.

■ Desserts—a Low-GI Finish ■

It's fairly easy to get at least one low-GI food into your dinner through dessert. This is because so many of the basic components of dessert, like fruit and dairy products, are low GI. Desserts can make a valuable contribution to our fruit and dairy intake—foods that are often underconsumed, even by healthy eaters. What's more, desserts are usually rich in carbohydrate, which means they add to our feelings of satiety, helping to signify the completion of eating.

A word about sugar in desserts: as we've noted, sugar, a common ingredient in traditional desserts, has a moderate GI (GI = 60)—and most sugary foods have low to moderate GI values. Cakes and cookies made with or without sugar have similar GI values. Recipes incorporating fruit for sweetness rather than sugar may have more fiber and lower GI values. Remember, fruits such as apples, pears, peaches, nectarines, plums, cherries, and berries tend to have the lowest GI.

Delicious low-GI dessert basics

Citrus. These winter fruits are an excellent source of vitamin C. Soak segments of a variety of citrus fruits in orange juice with a dash of brandy, scatter with raisins, and serve as winter fruit salad.

Cherries. With a GI of 63, cherries are intermediate GI, so you should watch your portions. Serve cherries around a dollop of low-fat plain yogurt drizzled with honey. Add a sprinkling of ground flaxseeds to increase your day's omega-3 intake.

Stone fruits. Apricots, peaches, plums, and nectarines at farmers' markets or in the grocery store signal the beginning of warmer weather. Fresh sliced peaches or nectarines are delicious with ice cream or yogurt. Sprinkle fresh peach halves with cinnamon or nutmeg and try them lightly grilled.

Pears and apples. At their peak during autumn and winter, these are available in most places all year. To prepare, simply wash and slice—or grill or bake. However you serve them, they provide the perfect finish to a meal.

Grapes. One of the most popular fruits with children, because they are so sweet and easy to eat (especially the seedless varieties). Put a bowl on the table after a meal, include them in a fruit salad, or freeze them for a fun snack.

Custard, pudding, ice cream, and yogurt. Look for low-fat varieties for a cool and creamy accompaniment to your fruit.

■ Eight Quick and Easy ■
Low-GI Dessert Ideas

1. Combine a pint of washed, hulled, and halved strawberries with a tablespoon of sugar in a small saucepan. Stir over medium heat for about 5 minutes until the strawberries soften and a syrup forms. Serve warm or chilled over low-fat vanilla ice cream.
2. Remove the core from large green apples and stuff with a combination of raisins, chopped dried apricots, cinnamon, and a teaspoon of brown sugar. Serve with low-fat plain yogurt or vanilla pudding.
3. Drain a can of peaches. Spoon into bowls. Pour some low-fat pudding over the peaches, then stir in crumbled coconut macaroons.
4. Make a fruit crisp by topping cooked fruit with a mixture of toasted oats, wheat flakes, a little melted butter or margarine, and honey.
5. Slice a firm banana in half lengthwise and top with 2 scoops of light vanilla ice cream. Spoon fresh fruit puréed in a food processor over the top and sprinkle with toasted almonds.
6. Top unsweetened canned fruit halves with a combination of shredded coconut, brown sugar, and cinnamon. Drizzle with a little of the juice from the can, then bake for 10 minutes till browned.
7. Brush 4–5 layers of phyllo pastry with low-fat milk (in place of butter or margarine). Place stewed or canned apple, raisins, currants, and mixed spice down the center and wrap as for a strudel. Brush the top with milk and bake in a hot oven for 15 minutes.

8. Lay a selection of sliced fresh fruits (e.g., mango, pineapple, strawberries, kiwi, or cantaloupe) on a platter and serve with a cup of plain low-fat yogurt combined with a tablespoon of honey.

■ Snacks— ■
Making the Right Between-Meal Choices

As we explained in "This for That" in chapter 6 (see page 80), because frequent small meals stimulate your metabolic rate, people who graze properly—eating small amounts of nutritious food throughout the day at frequent intervals—may actually be doing themselves a favor. Some satisfying snack ideas:

- smoothie made with with low-fat yogurt, milk, and a soft fruit, such as strawberries, cantaloupe, or banana
- cinnamon-raisin toast
- a juicy orange
- a bunch of grapes
- sourdough English muffin with jam
- a 6-ounce container of low-fat yogurt
- a can of unsweetened applesauce or diced peaches
- a glass of milk
- dried apricots
- a handful of raisins
- a big green apple
- a scoop of light ice cream in a cone

For something salty or strong tasting, try:

- baked tortilla chips and salsa
- hummus (process a can of chickpeas with 2 cloves of garlic, 2 tablespoons of tahini, and 2 tablespoons of lemon juice) with pumpernickel bread
- raw vegetables (baby carrots, green beans, pepper strips, radishes, celery, cucumber) with a low-fat dip, such as hummus

- a handful of wasabi chickpeas
- marinated vegetables, such as artichoke hearts, roasted peppers, or eggplant (blot off the oil on a paper towel), with toasted pita bread

▪15▪

Low-GI Eating
for Vegetarians

*I*f you're a vegetarian, you may be wondering: *Can I follow a low-GI diet and still get the nutrients and energy I need each day?* In a word, yes. In fact, the low-GI way of eating is ideally suited for vegetarians, who will find that they can easily incorporate the glycemic index into their lives.

As you probably know, many vegetarians tend to be healthy eaters who already consume a diet rich in low-GI foods, including legumes, whole grains, fruits, and vegetables. That's terrific, because there's now a wealth of scientific evidence to support the fact that a vegetarian diet can reduce the risk of heart disease, diabetes, and cancer. Unfortunately, many vegetarians also tend to have a diet that's too high in high-GI carbohydrates, saturated fat from dairy foods, and too low in heart-healthy omega-3's. The good news: a low-GI diet can provide you with the fuel you need to keep your body fueled, full of energy, and your metabolism running smoothly.

Vegetarians Tend to be Thinner than Meat Eaters

VEGETARIAN AND VEGAN women are less likely to be overweight than meat eaters, even taking into account age, exercise, and calorie intake, according to a recent study at Tufts University. Researchers surveyed 55,459 healthy middle-aged and older Swedish women about their eating habits, weight, and other health and lifestyle factors, and found that 40 percent of the women who said they ate meat, poultry, fish, eggs, and dairy products as well as plant-based foods were overweight or obese (a BMI of 25 or more), compared to 29 percent of the vegans. Vegetarians who ate dairy products but no meat, poultry, fish, or eggs were the leanest group, with 25 percent identified as being overweight or obese.

■ What Should Vegetarians Eat? ■

Building your diet around plant foods such as whole grains, legumes, fruits, vegetables, nuts, and seeds will provide you with all the nutrients you need for long-term health and well-being, not to mention plenty of protective, disease-fighting antioxidants and phytochemicals.

Protein. You're made of protein—your muscles, bones, skin, hair, and virtually every other body part are essentially protein, which consists of basic "building blocks" called amino acids. There are twenty different amino acids, and they can be found in many of the foods you eat. The body makes some amino acids on its own (these are called nonessential amino acids); but there are eight "essential" amino acids that your body *can't* make, and you need to get them from food. Because your body can't stockpile them from one day to the next as it does fat or carbs, you need a daily supply of protein-rich foods.

What are the best sources of protein? Because they don't eat red meat, chicken, or fish, getting enough protein can be a problem for many vegetarians. But with some careful planning, you can get the protein you need from plant proteins by eating plenty of legumes (beans, chickpeas, and lentils), foods rich in soy protein (such as tofu), cereal grains (especially whole grains), and nuts and seeds. It's even easier if you eat dairy foods and eggs. Read on to find out the best sources of protein in a well-balanced vegetarian diet.

Legumes. Whether you buy them dried or canned, beans such as kidney, cannellini, borlotti, black beans, and haricot beans—and even good old baked beans—are one of nature's nutritional powerhouse foods, which is why we recommend you eat them every day. First, they're a valuable source of protein for vegetarians and vegans; for example, 7 oz (200 g) of beans, lentils, or chickpeas provides an average of 15 grams of protein. Second, they're high in fiber and are an important source of carbs, B vitamins (including folate), minerals such as iron, zinc, and magnesium, and potent phytochemicals. They're versatile, too: you can add them to soups and salads, casseroles, and stir-fries, use them as a topping or filling, or make them into spreads, such as hummus.

Low-fat dairy foods. Dairy is another fantastic source of protein. Just 1 cup (8 fl oz) of skim milk, a 180-gram (6 oz) container of low-fat yogurt, or a 30-gram (1 oz) piece of low-fat cheddar cheese provide almost 10 grams of protein along with calcium, and vitamins A, B, and D. Keep in mind that not all dairy products contain calcium: butter doesn't, nor does cream or sour cream. Instead, they're primarily sources of unhealthy saturated fat.

Soybeans and soy products. Protein-rich soybeans have long been a staple of Asian diets, and thankfully, many people around the world are beginning to incorporate them into their diet. After all, just 210 grams (7 oz) of cooked or canned soybeans provides a whopping 24 grams of protein! Soybeans are also rich in fiber, iron, zinc, vitamin B, and phytochemicals. Though they're higher in fat than other legumes, the majority of the fat they contain is polyunsaturated. Plus, soy protein has also been found to help lower cholesterol levels in the blood. Soybeans are the basis of a variety of protein-rich products and meat substitutes, including tofu, tempeh, textured vegetable protein (TVP), and vegetarian sausages and burgers.

If you choose not to eat dairy products, some excellent nutritional equivalents are beverages, cheeses, yogurts, and desserts made from soy, and they're also low in saturated fat, cholesterol free, and rich in phytochemicals. However, soy products are not naturally high in calcium and can still be high in fat, so it's important to look for calcium-fortified varieties and to choose low-fat products—especially if you're watching your weight.

Nuts and seeds. A small handful of nuts can help you get the protein you need. For example, a 30-gram (1 oz) serving of most nuts provides around 5 grams protein (macadamias and pecans have less). Nuts are among the richest sources of the antioxidants vitamin E and selenium in our diet, but they are high in unsaturated fat and should be eaten in moderation. A small amount makes a healthy snack, a crunchy topping for salads, stir-fries, and desserts, or you can add nuts (whole or chopped) to muesli mixes, fillings, and stuffings.

Seeds such as sesame (and tahini, a paste of sesame seeds), pumpkin, sunflower, and flaxseeds also play a valuable role in the diet, and not only for their protein content. Just 15 grams (½ oz) provides about 3 to 4 grams protein along with iron, zinc, essential fatty acids and a range of vitamins, minerals, and antioxidants. Add them to muesli mixes, oatmeal, salads, and stir-fries.

Cereal grains. Grains are the seeds of cereal plants; they include barley, buckwheat, bulgur, maize, millet, oats, quinoa, rice, rye, spelt, and wheat. Whether you eat them as whole grains (such as brown rice or pearl barley), processed (such as white rice), or as one of the staple foods made from them (bread, breakfast cereals, pasta, noodles, and couscous), they can actually be good sources of protein and play an important role in vegetarian and vegan diets. Did you know that 1 cup (7½ oz) of cooked brown rice provides nearly 6 grams of protein, and a slice of mixed-grain bread or 30 grams (1 oz) of raw rolled oats around 3 grams? They are also the most concentrated sources of carbohydrates in our diet, and they're low in fat, packed with essential vitamins and minerals, and rich in fiber (provided you eat whole-grain varieties). Studies around the world show that eating plenty of whole grains reduces the risk of heart disease, type 2 diabetes, and certain types of cancer.

Wheat protein and seitan. A traditional food for Buddhists, seitan (pronounced SAY-tahn) is sometimes called "wheat meat." It comes from wheat gluten (the protein part of flour) and is an alternative to soy-based meat substitutes, such as tofu. It has a chewy texture and neutral taste, and tends to absorb the flavor of the foods you cook it with. Seitan is sold chilled in tubs or frozen in blocks, chunks, and strips. For best results when cooking, add it to dishes at the last minute, heating it just until it's warmed through.

How Much Protein Do You Need?

TO MAINTAIN YOUR body tissues and keep the engine in good repair you need around 40–55 grams (1½–2 oz) of protein a day—a lot less than many weight-loss diets promote—which is easily achievable with a well-balanced diet. On average, women need about 45 grams of protein a day (more, if they are pregnant, breast-feeding, or extremely active) and men about 55 grams.

Protein—the bottom line

- Eat a wide variety of protein foods every day to make sure you get all the essential amino acids you need.
- Stock your pantry with legumes, whole grains (such as grainy breads, muesli, brown rice, pearl barley, and rolled oats), nuts, and seeds (sesame seeds, tahini, and pumpkin seeds). They're good sources of protein *and* of key nutrients, including iron and zinc.

Fats. As we've stressed throughout this book, it's so important—for vegetarians and nonvegetarians alike—to know your fats. That means focusing on the good fats and giving the bad ones the boot.

A low-fat diet is not necessarily the only way to eat for overall health or even weight loss. In fact, your body needs a certain amount of good or unsaturated fat—think nuts, seeds, olive oil, and avocados— to function properly and thrive. Good fats:

▶ provide you with essential fatty acids
▶ help you absorb the fat-soluble vitamins A, D, E, and K
▶ form part of your body's hormones
▶ provide insulation
▶ help you absorb some antioxidants from fruit and vegetables
▶ help to make food taste better

Your body actually requires some types of fats—called essential fatty acids—that can't be manufactured by your body and have to be obtained through your diet. The best sources of these for vegetarians are polyunsaturated oils, flaxseeds and flaxseed oil, mustard seed oil, canola oil, nuts, and seeds.

The problem with fat is that it provides lots of calories—more than protein or carbs per gram. The main form in which our bodies store those extra calories is—you guessed it—fat. It's easy to reduce your fat intake when you know it's there (the most concentrated sources of fat in our diets are butter, margarines, and oils). But keep in mind that most snack foods, cakes, cookies, potato chips, muffins, regular popcorn, or a packet of instant noodles all contain a fair bit of fat as well. That's why it's important to read the label and to shop for products low in saturated fat, rather than just low-fat products. (The saturated-fat content should be less than 20 percent of the total fat.)

Go Easy on Cheese

CHEESE CAN BE a major source of saturated fat in vegetarian diets; all too often a cheesy dish is the only vegetarian option on the restaurant menu. But most cheese is around 30 percent fat, most of it saturated. So opt for low-fat choices such as ricotta or cottage cheese for your everyday cheese choice.

Healthy fats and oils include:

- Olive, peanut and canola oils
- Mustard seed, avocado, rice bran, and macadamia oils
- Flaxseed oil (can't be heated)
- Soft margarines and spreads made with olive, canola, sunflower, or other seed oils
- Avocados, olives
- Soybeans
- Almonds, brazil nuts, cashews, hazelnuts, macadamias, pistachio nuts, peanuts, and walnuts
- Flaxseeds, sunflower seeds, pumpkin seeds, sesame seeds
- Nut and seed spreads, such as peanut butter, almond spread, or tahini
- Muesli (untoasted)

Bad fats include:

- Full cream (full fat) dairy products—milk, cream, sour cream, cream cheese, cheese, ice cream
- Coconut and palm oils
- Ghee, solid frying oils, and margarines
- Potato chips, packaged snacks
- Cakes, cookies, pastries, pies, pizza
- Deep-fried foods-chips, spring rolls, tempura, battered foods

How Much Fat Do You Need?

NOT MUCH. UNLESS you are a very active person, 2–4 servings a day is all you need. One serving is equivalent to:

- 2 teaspoons of monounsaturated or polyunsaturated oil or margarine
- 1 tablespoon of oil-based vinaigrette
- 15 grams (½ oz) of nuts
- 40 grams (1½ oz) of avocado

Polyunsaturated fats are made up of omega-3 and omega-6 fats—and the balance between these is important for good health. Since vegetarians tend to consume more omega-6 and less omega-3, focus on including foods that are specifically sources of omega-3, such as walnuts, flaxseeds, soy products, or flaxseed oil. When preparing meals, try using a variety of different oils, depending on the dish—monounsaturated oil, such as canola or olive oil, is a good idea for cooking, as these oils are both "omega-neutral," meaning they will not worsen the balance of omega-6's and omega-3's.

Fats—the bottom line

- Focus on the good fats.
- Choose low-fat dairy products.
- Be aware of the hidden fats in snack foods.
- Stock your pantry with nuts and seeds that are good sources of omega-3.

Carbohydrates

As we've discussed throughout this book, carbs are a vital source of energy, and help you function at your best. Some foods contain a large amount of carbohydrate (cereals, potatoes, sweet potatoes, legumes, and corn are good examples), while others, such as string beans, broccoli, and salad greens, have very small amounts of carbohydrate. Breast milk, cow's milk, and milk products also contain carbohydrate in the form of milk sugar, or lactose.

What are the best sources?

Vegetarian and vegan diets tend to be high in carbohydrates (and fiber, too) because they are plant-based. Because of that, vegetarians especially need to pay attention to the quality of the carbohydrates they're consuming. Below are good sources of healthy, low-GI carbohydrates.

Grains. Cereal grains such as barley, buckwheat, bulgur, maize, millet, oats, quinoa, rice, rye, spelt, and wheat, and the enormous variety of foods made from them, including bread, breakfast cereals, pasta, noodles, and couscous, are the richest sources of carbohydrates. They also provide you with fiber and protein and many vitamins and minerals, especially if you choose whole-grain foods.

Each of the following servings will give you between 20 and 30 grams of carbohydrate:

- 2 slices of bread
- 1 cup of breakfast cereal
- ½ cup of rolled oats or muesli
- ½ cup of cooked rice or other small grains, such as bulgur or cracked wheat
- 1 cup of cooked pasta, noodles or couscous

Legumes. These are probably the second-richest source of carbohydrates in a vegetarian diet (1 cup of cooked or canned beans, chickpeas or lentils provides between 20 and 30 grams of carbohydrate), as well as being a major source of protein, vitamin B, iron, and zinc.

Vegetables. The higher-carbohydrate vegetables are the starchy ones that grow under the ground—potato, taro, yam, and sweet potato (2 small potatoes or half a medium sweet potato, for example, will provide 20 to 30 grams of carbohydrate). Parsnip, beet, pumpkin, carrot, turnips, and peas also provide adequate amounts of carbohydrates. Corn, while strictly a grain, is also high in carbohydrates (1 cup of kernels or a cob of corn will provide 20 to 30 grams of carbohydrate). Most other vegetables are low in carbohydrate, but are often valuable sources of vitamins and minerals along with protective antioxidants, so be sure to include them in your diet.

Fruit. A high fruit and vegetable intake has been consistently linked with better health (as have vegetarian diets)—perhaps because fruits and vegetables are packed with antioxidants. Fruit will also contribute to your carbohydrate intake (in the form of fruit sugars) but doesn't provide nearly as much carbohydrate as the cereal grains. Dried fruits are an exception, with many being as high in carbohydrate as cereal grains (a 30 g/1 oz serving provides between 10 and 20 grams of carbohydrate), and they are also a concentrated source of many vitamins and minerals.

Low-fat dairy foods and soy alternatives. Don't overlook calcium-rich dairy foods as a source of carbohydrates. Consuming 1 cup (8 fl oz) of low-fat or skim milk will provide you with about 12 grams of carbohydrate. Notably, soy beverages do not contain lactose, but generally contain the sugar sucrose; as a result, 1 cup contains around 15 grams of carbohydrate. (Be sure to look for the low-fat, calcium-enriched varieties.) Dairy products, including yogurt, custard, and ice cream (and the soy equivalents), are also good sources of carbohydrate, but cheese is not.

How Much Carbohydrate Do You Need?

SEE CHAPTER 5, which is devoted to exactly this question.

■ Why Choose Low-GI Carbohydrates ■

Eating a lot of high-GI foods can be detrimental to your health, because it pushes your body to extremes. This is especially true if you are overweight and sedentary. In the same way that the storm drain pipes of a city are pushed to the limit after a heavy downpour, your body's glucose response mechanisms are stretched after a load of quickly digested carbohydrates. In order to prevent this, you should replace highly refined starchy carbohydrate foods like most breads, processed breakfast cereals, cookies, and crackers with less processed carbohydrates like whole cereal grains, fruits, legumes, and vegetables.

Eating more low-GI carbs:

- reduces your insulin levels
- lowers your cholesterol levels
- helps control your appetite
- halves your risk of heart disease and diabetes
- means you are eating foods closer to the way nature intended

Carbohydrates—the bottom line

To ensure that you are eating enough carbohydrates, and the right kind, you should eat:

▶ fruits or vegetables at every meal, or for snacks
▶ at least one low-GI food at each meal
▶ lots of fiber-rich whole grains

Healthy low-GI vegetarian guidelines

Every day:

▶ Eat seven or more servings of fruit and vegetables (ideally, five servings of vegetables and two servings of fruit).
▶ Make the most of whole-grain breads and cereals with a low GI.
▶ Include a variety of plant proteins.
▶ Make sure you eat a handful of nuts regularly.
▶ Choose low-fat dairy products or calcium-enriched alternatives.
▶ Opt for monounsaturated and omega-3 polyunsaturated fats, such as olive and canola oil, and those found in nuts, seeds, and avocado.

In addition to the vegetarian recipes you'll find among the more than forty-five recipes in chapter 17, we also encourage you to consult *The New Glucose Revolution Low GI Vegetarian Cooking*, which includes eighty delicious vegetarian and vegan recipes.

·16·

Cooking the Low-GI Way

To make it easy to cook the low-GI way every day, at every meal, you need to stock the right foods. Here are some ideas for what to keep in your pantry, fridge, and freezer—and on the countertop.

■ What to Keep in Your Pantry ■

- **Asian sauces:** Hoisin, oyster, soy, and fish sauces are a good basic range.
- **Barley:** One of the oldest cultivated cereals, barley is very nutritious and high in soluble fiber. Look for products such as pearl barley to use in soups, stews, and pilafs.
- **Black pepper:** Buy freshly ground pepper or grind your own peppercorns.
- **Bread:** Low-GI options include grainy, stone-ground whole-grain, pumpernickel, sourdough, English muffins, flat bread, and pita bread. Choose breads that are made with intact kernals.

- **Breakfast cereals:** These include traditional rolled or steel-cut oats, natural muesli, and low-GI packaged breakfast cereals.
- **Bulgur wheat:** Use it to make tabbouli, or add to vegetable burgers, stuffings, soups, and stews.
- **Canned beans:** Canned beans of all varieties, chickpeas, and lentils are now widely available and are convenient to use and a great time-saver. See also dried beans, below.
- **Canned evaporated skim milk:** Makes an excellent substitution for cream in pasta sauce.
- **Canned fish:** Keep a good stock of canned tuna packed in spring water, and canned sardines, salmon, and crabmeat.
- **Canned vegetables:** Sweet corn kernels and tomatoes can help to boost the vegetable content of a meal. Tomatoes, in particular, can be used freely, because they are rich in antioxidants, as well as having a low GI.
- **Couscous:** Ready in minutes; serve it with casseroles, stews, or stir-fries.
- **Curry pastes:** A tablespoon or so makes a delicious curry base
- **Dried beans and lentils:** Lentils, split peas, beans, chickpeas, and beans of all varieties (cannellini, butter, cranberry, kidney, pinto, lima, mixed, baked) all have low GI values and are very nutritious. Incorporate them in a recipe, perhaps as a partial substitution for meat, and try a vegetarian dish (such as chickpea curry, hummus, red lentil soup, Mexican burritos, or a bean salad) at least once a week. Some dry legumes can be cooked quickly—split red lentils, for example, take only twenty or so minutes to cook.
- **Dried fruits:** Dried apricots, fruit medley, raisins, prunes, and berries.
- **Dried herbs and spices:** Oregano, basil, thyme, parsley, rosemary, marjoram, ginger, garlic, hot peppers are most commonly used either fresh or dried.
- **Honey:** Try to avoid the commercial honeys or honey blends, and use the "pure" honey, locally harvested, if possible. These varieties have a much lower GI naturally.
- **Jam:** A tablespoon of good-quality jam (with no added sugar) contains fewer calories than lightly spreading butter or margarine on toast.

- **Mustard:** Seeded or whole-grain mustard is useful as a sandwich spread, in salad dressings and sauces.
- **Noodles:** Many Asian noodles, such as Hokkien, udon, and rice vermicelli, have low to intermediate GI values because of their dense texture, whether they are made from wheat or rice flour.
- **Nuts:** Try a handful of nuts (about 1 ounce) every other day. Also, try adding soy "nuts" (dry roasted soy beans) and/or Chick Nuts (see recipe on page 258) to a nut mix.
- **Oils:** Try olive oil for general use; some extra-virgin olive oil for salad dressings, marinades, and dishes that benefit from its flavor; and sesame oil for Asian-style stir-fries. Canola or olive oil cooking sprays are handy, too.
- **Pasta:** A food to be eaten as often as desired—just remember to stick with moderate portions. Fresh or dried, the preparation is easy. Simply boil in water until just tender or al dente, drain, and toss with pesto, a tomato sauce, or a sprinkle of Parmesan, pepper, and olive oil. Pasta is also rich in B vitamins.
- **Quinoa:** This whole grain cooks in about 10 to 15 minutes and has a slightly chewy texture. It can be used as a substitute for rice, couscous, or bulgur wheat. It is very important to rinse the grains thoroughly before cooking.
- **Rice:** Basmati rice or Uncle Ben's converted long-grain rice are good choices, because they have a lower GI than, for example, jasmine rice.
- **Rolled oats:** Besides their use in oatmeal, oats can be added to cakes, cookies, breads, and desserts.
- **Sea salt:** Use in moderation.
- **Spices:** Most spices, including ground cumin, turmeric, cinnamon, paprika, and nutmeg, should be bought in small quantities, because they lose pungency with age and incorrect storage.
- **Stock:** Make your own stock or buy ready-made products that are available in long-life cartons in the supermarket. To keep the sodium content down with ready-made stocks, look out for a low-salt option.
- **Tomato paste:** Can be used with great versatility in soups, sauces, and casseroles.
- **Vinegar:** White-wine vinegar, red-wine vinegar, and balsamic vinegar are excellent for salads. A vinaigrette dressing (1

tablespoon of vinegar and 2 teaspoons of oil) with your salad can lower the blood glucose response to the whole meal by up to 30 percent. You may use lemon juice instead of vinegar.

■ What to Keep in Your Refrigerator ■

▶ **Bacon:** Bacon is a flavorful ingredient in many dishes. You can make a little bacon go a long way by trimming off all fat and chopping it finely. Lean ham is often a more economical and leaner way to go. In casseroles and soups, a ham or bacon bone imparts a fine flavor without much fat (but it's also fine to leave out of a recipe that calls for one if you're vegetarian).

▶ **Bottled vegetables:** Sundried tomatoes, olives, grilled eggplant, and peppers are handy to keep as flavorful additions to pastas and sandwiches.

▶ **Capers, olives, and anchovies:** These can be bought in jars and kept in the refrigerator once opened. They are tasty (but salty) additions to pasta dishes, salads, sauces, and pizzas.

▶ **Cheese:** Any reduced-fat cheese is great to keep handy in the fridge. A block of Parmesan is indispensable and will keep for up to a month. Reduced-fat cottage and ricotta cheeses have a short life, so are best bought as needed, and they can be a good alternative to butter or margarine in a sandwich.

▶ **Condiments:** Keep jars of minced garlic, chile, or ginger in the refrigerator to spice up your cooking in an instant.

▶ **Eggs:** To enhance your intake of omega-3 fats, we suggest using omega-3-enriched eggs. Although the yolk is high in cholesterol, the fat in eggs is predominantly monounsaturated and is therefore considered a "good fat."

▶ **Fish:** Seafood is generally a healthy choice, but salmon, anchovies, mackerel, trout, herrings, and sardines are richest in beneficial omega-3 fatty acids. Include fish at least once a week. Today most fish stores sell a wide variety of fresh fish, which you can use immediately or freeze for later use.

▶ **Fresh herbs:** Even if you have a cupboard full of dried herbs and spices, fresh herbs are available in most supermarkets (or easily grown at home in pots, window boxes, or gardens); there really is no substitute for the flavor they impart. For variety try parsley, basil, mint, chives, thyme, oregano, rosemary, and cilantro.

▶ **Fresh fruit:** Almost all fruits make an excellent low-GI snack. When they're in season, try fruit such as apples, oranges, pears, grapes, grapefruit, peaches, apricots, strawberries, and mangoes. Stonefruits and manos are best not refrigerated.

▶ **Lemons/lemon juice:** Try a fresh squeeze with ground black pepper on vegetables rather than butter. The lemon juice's acidity slows gastric emptying and lowers the GI value of a food. Bottled juice is now also widely available in the refrigerator case at supermarkets. You can also find fresh lemon juice in plastic squeeze bottles with the fresh lemons. (Some bottles look like lemons!)

▶ **Meat:** Lean varieties are better—try lean beef, lamb fillets, pork fillets, chicken (breast or drumsticks), and ground beef.

▶ **Milk:** Skim or low-fat milk is best, or try low-fat calcium-enriched soy milk.

▶ **Vegetables:** Keep on hand a variety of seasonal vegetables, such as spinach, broccoli, cauliflower, Asian greens, asparagus, zucchini, and mushrooms. Peppers, scallions, and sprouts (mung bean and snowpea sprouts) can be used to bulk up a salad. Sweet corn, sweet potato, and yam are essential to your low-GI food store.

▶ **Yogurt:** Low-fat natural yogurt provides the most calcium for the fewest calories. Have vanilla or fruit versions as a dessert, or use natural yogurt as a condiment in savory dishes.

■ What to Keep in Your Freezer ■

▶ **Frozen berries:** Berries can make any dessert special, and by using frozen ones it means you don't have to wait until berry season in order to indulge. Try blueberries, raspberries, and strawberries.

▶ **Frozen yogurt:** This is a fantastic substitute for ice cream, and some products even have a similar creamy texture, but with much less fat.

▶ **Frozen vegetables:** Keep a package of peas, beans, corn, spinach, or mixed vegetables in the freezer—these are handy to add to a quick meal.

▶ **Ice cream:** Reduced- or low-fat ice cream is ideal for a quick dessert, served with fresh fruit.

▪ What to Keep on the Kitchen Counter ▪

▶ **Tomatoes:** All that applies to tomato sauces and pastes applies to fresh tomatoes—which are especially enjoyable at the height of summer, when a wide range of fresh varieties (heirlooms, cherries, plums, and beefsteaks) are widely available. Tomatoes should never be refrigerated.

Making Sense of Food Labeling

FOOD LABELS CARRY considerable information today, but unfortunately, very few people know how to interpret them correctly. Often the claims on the front of the package don't mean quite what you think. Here are some prime examples:

- ▪ **Cholesterol free**—Be careful: the food may still be high in fat.
- ▪ **Reduced fat**—But is it low fat? Compare fat per 100 grams between products.
- ▪ **No trans fat**—But check the ingredient list for "hydrogenated or partially hydrogenated oil." FDA regulations allow up to 0.5 grams of it to count as zero trans fat—and the servings can add up.
- ▪ **No added sugar**—Do you realize it could still raise your blood glucose?
- ▪ **Lite or Light**—Light in what? FDA regulations specify that these can mean that a nutritionally altered product contains one-third fewer calories or half the fat of the standard version—and if the food derives 50 percent or more of its calories from fat, the reduction must be 50 percent of the fat. They could also mean simply

light in color or texture—in which case qualifying information needs to be included, though exceptions are made for foods like light brown sugar that have a long history of use.

To get the hard facts on the nutritional value of a food, look at the Nutrition Information table. Here you'll find the details regarding the fat, calorie, carbohydrate, fiber, and sodium content of the food. Here are the key points to look for:

- **Calories**—This is a measure of how much energy we get from a food. For a healthy diet we need to eat more foods with a low energy density and combine them with smaller amounts of higher-energy foods. To assess the energy density look at the calories per 100 grams. A low energy density is < 120 cals /100 grams.
- **Fat**—We want a low saturated fat content, ideally < 20 percent of the total fat. This means that if the total fat content is 10 grams, you want saturated fat < 2 grams. Strictly speaking, a food can be labeled as low in saturated fat if it contains < 1.5 grams saturated fat/100 grams.
- **Total carbohydrate**—This is the starch, fiber, and any naturally occurring and added sugars in the food. The *available carbohydrate* is the total carbohydrate − fiber. (There's no need to look at the sugar figure separately since it's the total carbohydrate that affects your blood glucose level.) You can use this figure if you are monitoring your carbohydrate intake and to calculate the glycemic load (GL) of your serving of the food. The GL = grams of available carbohydrate per serving × GI ÷100.
- **Fiber**—Most of us don't get enough fiber in our diet, so it's better to look for high-fiber foods. A high-fiber food contains > 3 grams of fiber per serving.
- **Sodium**—This is a measure of the nasty part of salt in our food. Our bodies need some salt, but most people consume much more than they need. Canned foods in particular tend to be high in sodium. Check the sodium content per 100 grams next time you buy— a low-sodium food contains less than 140 mg sodium/100 g.

·17·

More than 45
Low-GI Recipes

$\mathcal{T}$he following recipes are quick, delicious, low GI, and extreme-ly easy to make. They are full of healthy ingredients, such as whole grains, lean meats, fish and seafood, legumes, and fresh fruits and vegetables. The recipes reflect the *New Glucose Revolution* phi-losophy and emphasize:

- Low-GI carbs
- Monounsaturated and omega-3 fats
- A moderate to high level of protein

■ A Note About the Recipes ■
in this Book

All the recipes in this section have been analyzed using a computer-ized nutrient-analysis programs*, and the energy, protein, carbohy-

* Foodworks™, Xyris Software (Australia) Pty Ltd. and ESHA Food Processor SQL

drate, fat, and fiber content per serving are shown. If the recipe is rich in particular micronutrients, we have identified them for you.

We also identify each recipe as low, moderate, or high—both for GI and for GL. Where the recipe has a high GL, we suggest serving it with foods that have little glycemic impact, such as salads, vegetables, and protein—foods such as lean meat or seafood.

GI RATING

Low GI = 55 or less

Moderate GI = 56–69

High GI = 70 or more

The following information will help put this nutritional profile into context for you. Where a range of servings is given for the recipe, the nutritional information relates to the higher number.

GI—We have given each recipe a GI rating, which is our best estimate of the range in which the GI value falls. A calculated GI value is not realistic for all recipes, because the carbohydrate may be used in the recipe in a different form from that in which the original GI value of the food was tested.

Energy—This is a measure of how many calories a serving provides. A moderately active woman aged 18 to 54 years requires about 1,900 calories a day; a man, about 2,400 calories. Those who burn lots of energy through exercise need a higher calorie intake than those who live more sedentary lives.

Carbohydrate—It is not necessary to calculate how many grams of carbohydrate you eat on a daily basis; however, if you're an athlete or you have diabetes, you may find this information useful. To consume around 50 percent of energy from carbohydrate, on average, women need about 200 grams a day, while men need about 300 grams. Athletes can consume anywhere from 300 to 700 grams of carbohydrate a day, providing 50 to 60 percent of their energy needs. To have an idea of the impact the carbohydrate in the recipe may have on your blood-sugar level and insulin response, multiply the carbohydrate content per serving of the recipe by its GI value to give you the glycemic load. See pages 16–18 for a discussion of the glycemic load and the tables in part 5 for glycemic load values.

Fat—We have aimed to keep our recipes low in fat, in particular low in saturated fat. For this reason we have used mono- and polyunsaturated margarines and oils. Omega-3 fatty acids from fish and seafood have many health benefits, so we have included a number of recipes containing these foods and used omega-3-enriched eggs.

The amount of fat that is appropriate in your diet depends on your calorie intake and the overall composition of your diet. A low-fat diet for most people could contain somewhere between 30 and 60 grams of fat per day. If you are not trying to lose weight, there is no harm in consuming larger amounts of fat, so long as it is predominantly unsaturated and has no added trans fat.

Fiber—Most of the recipes are high in fiber, both soluble and insoluble. Dietary guidelines recommend a daily fiber intake of at least 25 grams. People with diabetes should aim for 25 to 30 grams of fiber, as the American Diabetes Association recommends. A slice of wholewheat bread provides 2 grams of fiber, an average apple 4 grams. The average American consumes only about 11 grams of fiber a day.

So, that's the nutrition part of it. Now it's time to start cooking and embark on the low-GI road to fitness and good health. Enjoy!

Breakfasts
and Brunches

■

Honey Banana Smoothie

Peach Mango Raspberry Shake

Raisin-Studded Oatmeal

Muesli with Mixed Fresh Fruit

Buttermilk Pancakes with Glazed Fruit

Blueberry Muffins

Bran Muffins with Apples and Walnuts

Blueberry Oatmeal-Cornmeal Quick Bread

Red Pepper Spanish Tortilla

HONEY BANANA SMOOTHIE

The "smoothie"—a quick but sustaining breakfast. Many variations are possible using different combinations of fruits, milks, and yogurts. A COOK'S NOTE: The evaporated milk must be chilled to froth up well in this recipe.

PREPARATION TIME: 5 minutes ■ **COOKING TIME:** None ■ **SERVES 2**

---

1 large, ripe banana

1 tablespoon All-Bran breakfast cereal

1 cup low-fat milk, chilled

½ cup evaporated low-fat milk, well chilled

2 teaspoons honey

few drops vanilla extract

1. Peel banana and coarsely chop.
2. Combine with remaining ingredients in a blender and blend for 30 seconds or until smooth and thick. Serve immediately.

▶ LOW GI

PER SERVING:

CAL	190
CARB	35 g
FAT	0.5 g
FIBER	2 g

PEACH MANGO RASPBERRY SHAKE

*P*eaches, mangoes, and raspberries are all low-GI fruits, making this a great choice for breakfast.

PREPARATION TIME: 5 minutes ■ **COOKING TIME:** None ■ **SERVES** 1

¼ cup chopped fresh or frozen peaches

¼ cup chopped fresh or frozen mango

¼ cup fresh or frozen raspberries

¼ cup non-fat plain yogurt

½ cup apple juice

1. Combine all ingredients in a blender and puree until smooth. Serve immediately.

> **▶ LOW GI**
>
> **PER SERVING:**
>
> | CAL | 170 |
> |------|------|
> | CARB | 39 g |
> | FAT | 0 g |
> | FIBER | 5 g |

RAISIN-STUDDED OATMEAL

A quick and easy breakfast with a lot of stick-to-your-ribs character.

PREPARATION TIME: 5 minutes ■ COOKING TIME: 10 minutes ■ SERVES 2

⅔ cup rolled oats

1 cup low-fat milk, approximately

1 small ripe banana, mashed

1 heaping tablespoon raisins

▶ LOW GI

PER SERVING:

CAL	210
CARB	38 g
FAT	3 g
FIBER	3 g

1. Place the oats in a saucepan or large microwaveable bowl. Add sufficient water to cover, plus about ⅔ cup of the milk.
2. Bring to a boil and boil for 2 minutes or microwave on high for 1 to 2 minutes.
3. Add the banana and cook 1 to 2 minutes more.
4. Add the remaining milk to make a smooth consistency and stir in raisins.

MUESLI WITH MIXED FRESH FRUIT

*C*reamy rolled oats, plump raisins, and crunchy almonds combined with plain yogurt, milk, and fresh fruit.

PREPARATION TIME: 5 minutes ■ SOAKING TIME: overnight
■ COOKING TIME: None ■ SERVES 2

---

1 cup rolled oats

⅔ cup low-fat milk

1 tablespoon raisins

½ cup (4 oz) low-fat plain yogurt

¼ cup whole almonds, chopped

1 apple, grated

lemon juice (optional)

mixed fresh fruit, such as strawberries, pear, plum, blueberries, cherries

1. Combine the oats, milk, and raisins in a bowl. Cover and refrigerate overnight.
2. Add the yogurt, almonds, and apple; mix well.
3. To serve, adjust the flavor with lemon juice. Serve with fresh fruit.

▶ LOW GI

PER SERVING:

CAL	365
CARB	50 g
FAT	11 g
FIBER	6 g

BUTTERMILK PANCAKES
WITH GLAZED FRUIT

*G*olden light pancakes served with warm, soft summer fruits. A COOK'S NOTE: Dried-fruit medley is a mixture of dried fruit and is available from supermarkets and health-food stores.

PREPARATION TIME: 1 hour 20 minutes ▪ **COOKING TIME:** 25 minutes ▪ **SERVES** 4

---

1 cup 1-minute oats or unprocessed oat bran

2 cups buttermilk

½ cup dried-fruit medley, chopped

½ cup white flour, sifted

2 teaspoons sugar

1 teaspoon baking soda

1 egg, lightly beaten

2 teaspoons mono-or polyunsaturated margarine, melted

low-fat milk (optional)

Glazed fruit

1 tablespoon mono-polyunsaturated margarine

1 tablespoon brown sugar

6 medium peaches or apricots or nectarines

> ▶ **LOW GI**
>
> **PER SERVING:**
>
> | | |
> |---|---|
> | CAL | 420 |
> | CARB | 60 g |
> | FAT | 12 g |
> | FIBER | 6 g |

1. Combine the oats and buttermilk in a bowl and let stand 10 minutes.

2. Stir in the dried fruit, flour, sugar, baking soda, egg, and margarine; mix thoroughly. Let stand for about 1 hour.

3. After standing, add a little low-fat milk if the mixture is too thick.

4. Heat a nonstick frying pan or griddle and spray with cooking spray or grease lightly with margarine. Pour in about 3 tablespoons of batter, cook over medium-high heat until bubbly on top and lightly browned underneath. Turn pancake to brown on other side.

5. Repeat with remaining batter.

6. Set aside to keep warm.

7. To make the glazed fruit, melt the margarine and sugar together over medium heat in frying pan. Stir until sugar is dissolved. Add the sliced fruit and cook over medium heat 2–3 minutes until softened. Serve warm over the pancakes.

BLUEBERRY MUFFINS

*Y*ou can substitute the blueberries with any berries in this recipe, such as raspberries. These muffins freeze well and make a great snack to take to work or school.

PREPARATION TIME: 10 minutes ■ **COOKING TIME:** 20 minutes
■ **MAKES** 12 Muffins

---

1 cup blueberries

1½ cups rolled oats

½ cup unprocessed oat bran

1½ cups whole-wheat flour or whole-grain pastry flour

2½ teaspoons baking powder

¼ teaspoon salt

1 cup apple juice

3 tablespoons canola oil

⅓ cup honey

1 egg

▶ **MODERATE GI**

PER SERVING:

CAL	93
CARB	34 g
FAT	5 g
FIBER	4 g

1. Preheat oven to 350°F. Coat a 12-cup muffin pan with cooking spray or line with paper baking cups.

2. In a large mixing bowl, mix together the blueberries, oats, oat bran, flour, baking powder, and salt.

3. In another bowl, combine the apple juice, oil, honey, and egg. Add the flour mixture to the liquid mixture and stir until just combined.

4. Spoon the muffin mixture into the prepared pan, filling the cups three-quarters full. Bake for 15–20 minutes or until golden and cooked through. Cool for 10 minutes on a wire rack before removing from the pan.

BRAN MUFFINS WITH APPLES AND WALNUTS

*C*hopped fresh apples, not the usual applesauce, flavor these moist muffins. They are high in fiber and much lower in fat than traditional bran muffins.

PREPARATION TIME: 20 minutes ■ **COOKING TIME:** 15 minutes
■ **MAKES** 12 Muffins

---

3 tablespoons mono- or polyunsaturated margarine, softened

½ cup packed brown sugar

⅓ cup fat-free plain yogurt

3 tablespoons honey

1 egg

1 teaspoon grated orange peel

1¼ cups wheat bran

1 cup whole-wheat pastry flour or unbleached flour

1½ teaspoons baking soda

½ teaspoon salt

¼ teaspoon grated nutmeg

¼ teaspoon ground cinnamon

1 small apple, peeled, cored, and diced

¼ cup finely chopped walnuts

1. Preheat oven to 375°F. Coat a 12-cup muffin pan with cooking spray or line with paper baking cups.

2. Place the butter in a large bowl and beat with an electric mixer until smooth. Add the brown sugar and beat until creamy. Add the yogurt, honey, egg, and orange peel, beating after each addition.

3. In another bowl, combine the wheat bran, flour, baking soda, salt, nutmeg, and cinnamon.

4. Fold the flour mixture into the yogurt mixture, stirring just enough to incorporate the ingredients. Fold in the apples and walnuts.

5. Spoon the batter into the prepared muffin pan. Bake for 15 minutes, or until a toothpick inserted into the center of a muffin comes out clean. Remove from the pan and cool on a wire rack.

> ▶ **MODERATE GI**
>
> **PER SERVING:**
>
> | | |
> |---|---|
> | CAL | 148 |
> | CARB | 26 g |
> | FAT | 5 g |
> | FIBER | 4 g |

BLUEBERRY OATMEAL-CORNMEAL QUICK BREAD

*C*ookbook author and former innkeeper Crescent Dragonwagon developed this tender quick bread, which brings together in one bread ingredients familiar to every baker but unusually combined here (one doesn't often see cornmeal and rolled oats in the same recipe). This is wonderful served as part of breakfast or brunch.

PREPARATION TIME: 25 minutes ■ **COOKING TIME:** 40–50 minutes ■ **SERVES** 16

1½ cups unbleached all-purpose flour

⅓ cup stone-ground yellow cornmeal

½ teaspoon baking soda

1 teaspoon baking powder

½ teaspoon salt

2 cups fresh blueberries, washed and picked over, or thawed frozen blueberries

¼ cup old-fashioned rolled oats

2 to 4 tablespoons walnuts, toasted and chopped

3 tablespoons mild oil, (corn, canola, or peanut)

2 eggs

½ cup plus 2 tablespoons buttermilk

¾ cup sugar

Finely grated zest of 1 lemon or orange

▶ MODERATE GI

PER SERVING:

CAL	120
CARB	21 g
FAT	3 g
FIBER	1 g

1. Preheat oven to 350°F. Coat 4 mini-loaf pans with cooking spray. We like to bake it in mini-loaf pans, but you can also use 2 medium loaf pans.

2. Sift the flour, cornmeal, baking soda, baking powder, and salt together in a large bowl.

3. In a small bowl, combine the blueberries, oats, and walnuts. Sprinkle 1 tablespoon of flour mixture over them.

4. In a medium bowl, beat oil, eggs, buttermilk, sugar, and zest together.

5. Stir the wet mixture into the dry mixture using as few strokes as possible until a batter is formed.

6. Spoon batter into the prepared pans. Bake until lightly browned, about 40 to 50 minutes. Check two-thirds of the way through the baking period; if loaves are browning excessively, tent loosely with aluminum foil.

7. Let breads cool 10 minutes in pan, then run knife around the edges of the pan, and turn loaves out on a wire rack to cool completely.

RED PEPPER SPANISH TORTILLA

$\mathcal{D}$on't be confused by the name; Spanish tortillas are much closer to frittatas than to a flour tortilla (though unlike frittatas, they're not finished in the oven). This dish's higher GI potatoes, a classic ingredient in a Spanish tortilla, are married here with fresh or roasted red peppers, which have negligible carbohydrate. A side green salad with vinaigrette will help reduce the glycemic impact of the potatoes.

PREPARATION TIME: 10 minutes ■ COOKING TIME: 45 minutes ■ SERVES 8

---

6 tablespoons extra-virgin olive oil

2 large fresh or roasted red peppers, thinly sliced

1 onion, thinly sliced

6 small red potatoes, sliced

6 eggs, beaten

3 tablespoons chopped parsley

½ teaspoon salt

¼ teaspoon freshly ground black pepper

▶ MODERATE GI

PER SERVING:

CAL	161
CARB	11 g
FAT	14 g
FIBER	2 g

---

1. Heat 1 tablespoon of the oil in a large, nonstick skillet over medium heat. Add the peppers and onion and sauté, stirring often, for 10 minutes, or until browned and tender. Remove to a larger bowl.

2. Add 1 tablespoon of the remaining oil to the skillet, then add the potatoes. Cook, turning often, for 15 minutes, or until browned and tender. Remove to the bowl with the onion and red peppers.

3. Add the eggs, parsley, salt, and pepper to the bowl. Toss to mix well.

4. Wipe the skillet and add 2 tablespoons of the remaining oil. Pour the egg mixture into the pan. Place the pan over medium heat and cook, covered, for 15 minutes, or until the eggs start to set and the bottom browns.

5. Place a plate on top of the pan and invert the tortilla onto the plate. Add the remaining 2 tablespoons oil to the pan and slide the tortilla back into the pan. Cook for 5 minutes longer, or until browned. Allow to cool at room temperature and cut into 8 wedges to serve.

Soups, Salads and Vegetarian Sides

■

Lentil and Barley Soup

Minestrone Soup

Roasted Butternut Squash and White Bean Soup

Black Bean Soup

Spinach Salad with a Garlic Yogurt Dressing

Split Pea, Watercress and Goat Cheese Salad

Pasta and Red Bean Salad

LENTIL AND BARLEY SOUP

*B*oth lentils and barley are low-GI, and each with their distinctive flavors, contribute to make this zesty, satisfying winter soup a meal in itself.

PREPARATION TIME: 15 minutes ■ COOKING TIME: 1 hour ■ SERVES 4 to 6

---

1 tablespoon oil

1 large onion, finely chopped

2 cloves garlic, crushed, or 2 teaspoons minced garlic

½ teaspoon turmeric

2 teaspoons curry powder

½ teaspoon ground cumin

1 teaspoon minced hot peppers

6 cups water

1½ cups prepared vegetable or chicken stock

1 cup red lentils

½ cup pearl barley

1 15-ounce can tomatoes, undrained and crushed

salt

freshly ground black pepper

chopped fresh parsley or coriander, to serve

1. Heat the oil in a large saucepan. Add the onion, cover, and cook gently for about 10 minutes or until beginning to brown, stirring frequently.
2. Add the next 5 ingredients (garlic through hot peppers) and cook, stirring, for 1 minute.
3. Stir in the water, stock, lentils, barley, tomatoes, and salt and pepper to taste. Bring to a boil, cover, and simmer about 45 minutes or until the lentils and barley are tender.
4. Serve sprinkled with parsley or coriander.

▶ LOW GI

PER SERVING:

CAL	180
CARB	25 g
FAT	5 g
FIBER	5 g

MINESTRONE SOUP

*S*erve this hearty soup with true whole-grain bread and a green salad for a balanced and delicious low-GI meal.

PREPARATION TIME: 15 minutes ■ **COOKING TIME:** 1 hour 25 minutes ■ **SERVES 6**

---

1 15-ounce can cannellini beans, rinsed and drained

1 teaspoon olive oil

2 medium onions, chopped

2 cloves garlic, crushed

10 cups water

5 vegetable or beef bouillon cubes

3 carrots, diced

2 sticks celery, sliced

2 small zucchini, chopped

4 tomatoes (approximately 1 lb), diced

⅓ cup small macaroni pasta

2 tablespoons fresh parsley, chopped

freshly ground black pepper

grated Parmesan cheese, to serve (optional)

1. Heat a little oil in a large heavy-based saucepan. Add the onions and garlic and cook for about 5 minutes or until soft. Add the water, bouillon cubes, and drained beans. Bring to a boil.

2. Add the carrots, celery, zucchini, and tomatoes to the stock. Reduce heat and simmer, covered, for 1 hour.

3. Remove the lid and add the macaroni and stir. Continue to simmer for 10 to 15 minutes or until the macaroni is tender.

4. Stir in the parsley and add pepper to taste. Serve with Parmesan cheese.

▶ LOW GI

PER SERVING:

CAL	120
CARB	18 g
FAT	2 g
FIBER	7 g

ROASTED BUTTERNUT SQUASH AND WHITE BEAN SOUP

This is a quintessential autumn low-GI soup—perfect for gatherings of all types. The roasted squash and white beans readily soak up stock, so have plenty on hand to add as you need it. If you're not serving a crowd, this yields multiple lunches or dinners, and it freezes beautifully (freeze it in single-portion-size containers, which thaw more quickly than larger containers).

PREPARATION TIME: 45 minutes ■ **SOAKING TIME:** overnight
COOKING TIME: 2½ hours ■ **SERVES 8**

---

1 cup dried white beans
water
2–4 bay leaves

1 medium butternut squash (2–3 pounds)
1 head of garlic
olive oil
salt and freshly ground pepper

3 medium yellow onions
3 stalks celery
3 medium carrots
1 tablespooon olive oil
salt and freshly ground pepper
3 teaspoons dried thyme
6–8 cups vegetable stock
3 teaspoons ground cumin
¼ cup chopped fresh parsley and/or cilantro
¼ cup grated Parmesan cheese

1. Soak beans overnight in a large bowl of water, covered.
2. When you're ready to cook the beans, drain them, then bring to a boil in a medium saucepan, covered with water by about an inch. Once they boil, simmer for about an hour, with the lid ajar, or however long it takes for the beans to cook through. Keep an eye on the pot and add hot water as the water is absorbed by the beans. Cook just until the beans begin to fall apart. Set aside (with the bay leaves).
3. Slice the butternut squash in half lengthwise. Gently scoop out the pulp and seeds, scraping away only as much flesh as you need to clean out the pulp/seeds.
4. Fill the each of the two cavities with whole, unpeeled garlic cloves; generally, the number of cloves one medium head of garlic generates are just the right amount to fill, almost but not to overflowing, the two cavities. Lightly oil a heavy roasting pan (or heavy tray). Season the pan and the

squash halves with salt and freshly ground pepper. Carefully flip the squash halves, with the garlic cloves in the cavities, face down into the roasting pan (a metal spatula held over the cavities can help keep the cloves from spilling out, in the flip).

5. Roast in a 400-degree oven for about an hour—or until the skin is browned and crinkly, and the flesh is soft and easily pierced. Allow it to cool in the pan. Once it's cool, scoop out the squash flesh and pop the garlic cloves (which will soften/cook through, perfectly) and put through the medium or large disk of a food mill, or puree in a food processor. Set aside.

6. Finely dice the onions, celery, and carrots. Sauté in a large stockpot/soup pan over medium heat, starting first with the onions (about 10–15 minutes), then add the celery (for about 5 minutes), and then the carrots (about 10 minutes). Season with salt, pepper, and thyme. Add the butternut squash puree/mash, as well as the cooked white beans. Add about 4 cups of vegetable stock—or however much is necessary to cover the contents of the pot. Reduce heat to low and simmer. Add stock as necessary if the soup gets too thick. Soup can simmer on very low heat for 2–3 hours, but requires only about an hour or so if you don't have that much time. Shortly before serving, taste for seasoning and add, if necessary, a bit more salt, freshly ground pepper, a bit more thyme, and ground cumin.

■ Serve with a sprinkle of Parmesan and parsley or cilantro garnish.

▶ **LOW GI**

PER SERVING:

CAL	252
CARB	43 g
FAT	5 g
FIBER	12 g

BLACK BEAN SOUP

*B*eans are naturally a low-GI food and one of nature's nutritional power packs. They are considered good sources of protein, fiber, B vitamins, iron, zinc, and magnesium. Served with whole-grain bread and a salad, this makes a satisfying meal for a small crowd.

PREPARATION TIME: 25 minutes ■ SOAKING TIME: overnight
■ COOKING TIME: 1 hour 15 minutes ■ SERVES 6

---

1 cup dry black beans
½ cup diced onions
½ cup peeled and diced carrots
¼ cup diced celery
1 large red pepper, roasted
1 tablespoon minced fresh garlic
2 quarts vegetable stock
¼ teaspoon ground cumin
½ teaspoon salt
1 teaspoon chopped fresh oregano
2 teaspoons chopped fresh parsley
2 teaspoons chopped fresh cilantro

1. In a large bowl, cover black beans with 3½ cups water and soak overnight.
2. Rinse beans in a colander with fresh water and drain.
3. Lightly spray a large saucepan with olive oil. Sauté onions, carrots, celery, roasted pepper, and garlic. Add vegetable stock and black beans. Bring to a boil, reduce heat, and simmer for 1 hour.
4. When beans are tender, pour into a food processor and puree. Add cumin, salt, oregano, parsley, and cilantro. Serve with whole-grain bread.

▶ **LOW GI**

PER SERVING:

CAL	140
CARB	27 g
FAT	0.5 g
FIBER	5 g

SPINACH SALAD
WITH A GARLIC YOGURT DRESSING

*J*his makes delicious use of one of the classic salad greens and comes from Jane Frank's *Eating for Diabetes*, which, like the recipes in our New Glucose Revolution books provides GI ratings for its 125 recipes; this salad is low GI. Serve it with a low-GI truly whole-grain bread.

PREPARATION TIME: 15 minutes ■ COOKING TIME: none ■ SERVES 4

---

1 pound fresh spinach

2 tomatoes, peeled and diced

6 green onions, thinly sliced on the diagonal

5 tablespoons plain yogurt

2 tablespoons extra-virgin olive oil

2 garlic cloves, peeled and finely chopped

1 tablespoon fresh oregano leaves

sea salt and freshly ground pepper, to taste

1. Wash the spinach well in several changes of water. Dry the leaves carefully and tear into bite-size pieces. Place in a salad bowl together with the tomatoes and green onions.

2. Whisk together the yogurt, olive oil, chopped garlic, and oregano, and season to taste.

3. Toss the salad with the dressing and serve.

▶ **LOW GI**

PER SERVING:

CAL	124
CARB	11 g
FAT	8 g
FIBER	4 g

SPLIT PEA, WATERCRESS AND GOAT CHEESE SALAD

Created by Kate Tait for June 2006's *Delicious* magazine, this salad is a deliciously complete meal in itself and can be prepared, cooked, and served in around 30 minutes. You can buy roasted red peppers prepared in a jar; goat cheese is now available just about everywhere cheese is sold.

PREPARATION TIME: 15 minutes ■ **COOKING TIME:** 30 minutes ■ **SERVES** 4

---

1 cup green split peas, dry

1 tablespoon olive oil

juice of 1 lemon

2 teaspoons ground coriander

½ teaspoon ground ginger

1 red onion, very finely chopped

1 bunch watercress, stalks trimmed (3 cups sprigs)

2 roasted red peppers, cut into strips

¼ cup goat cheese

> ▶ **MODERATE GI**
>
> **PER SERVING:**
>
> | | |
> |---|---|
> | CAL | 273 |
> | CARB | 37 g |
> | FAT | 7 g |
> | FIBER | 13 g |

1. Cook the split peas in a saucepan of boiling water for 15–18 minutes until tender, but firm to the bite.

2. Meanwhile, make the dressing by placing the oil, lemon juice, spices, and onion in a large bowl and whisking until combined.

3. Drain the peas well and add to the dressing. Season to taste if desired and toss to combine. Stand for 10 minutes to let the flavors absorb, then toss with the watercress sprigs and red pepper strips.

4. Divide evenly among four plates and top with goat cheese.

PASTA AND RED BEAN SALAD

A summer salad full of flavor. Easy to prepare with canned beans.

PREPARATION TIME: 15 minutes ■ **COOKING TIME:** 15 minutes ■ **SERVES 4**

---

1 cup cooked pasta (e.g., shells, elbows, twists)

1 cup canned red kidney beans, well drained

3 green onions, finely chopped

1 tablespoon fresh parsley, finely chopped

Dressing

1 tablespoon olive oil

1 tablespoon wine vinegar

1 teaspoon Dijon mustard

1 clove garlic, crushed

freshly ground black pepper

1. Combine the pasta, beans, onions, and parsley in a serving bowl.
2. For the dressing, combine the oil, vinegar, mustard, garlic, and pepper in a screw-top jar; shake well to combine.
3. Pour the dressing over the pasta mixture and toss well.

▶ LOW GI

PER SERVING:

CAL	130
CARB	15 g
FAT	5 g
FIBER	4 g

Light Meals,
Lunches
and Savory Snacks

■

Sweet Corn and Crab Hotcakes with Arugula and Oven-roasted Tomatoes

Tabbouleh

Asian-style Scrambled Tofu

Asparagus, Arugula, and Lemon Barley "Risotto"

Whole Wheat Penne with Arugula and Edamame

Spicy Noodles

Pasta with Tangy Tomatoes

Chick Nuts

SWEET CORN AND CRAB HOTCAKES WITH ARUGULA AND OVEN-ROASTED TOMATOES

*I*nspired by Sydney, Australia, restaurateur Bill Granger, whose numerous restaurants have legions of fans, this recipe turns one of the sweetened breakfast staples of his original Bill's restaurant into a savory dinner dish. With its combo of crab and sweet corn, paired wth tomatos, it's perfect as an all-in-one, height-of-summer lunch or light supper.

PREPARATION TIME: 20 minutes ■ COOKING TIME: 55 minutes ■ SERVES 6

---

1 cup all-purpose flour

1 teaspoon baking powder

¼ teaspoon salt

¼ teaspoon paprika

2 eggs

½ cup milk

1 cup fresh corn kernels

1 cup lump crabmeat

⅔ cup roasted red peppers

½ cup shallots

¼ cup chopped cilantro and
  parsley, combined

4 tablespoons vegetable oil

To serve

1½ cups roasted tomatoes

1 bunch arugula

Olive oil

1. Sift flour, baking powder, salt, and paprika into a large bowl. Make a well in the center. In a separate bowl combine eggs and milk. Gradually add the egg mixture to the dry ingredients and whisk until you have a smooth, stiff batter.

2. Place corn, crabmeat, red peppers, shallots, cilantro, and parsley in a mixing bowl and add the flour batter to lightly bind the corn-crabmeat mixture.

3. Heat 2 tablespoons oil in a large, nonstick frying pan on medium heat. Drop ¼ cup batter into the pan, and repeat, making 2 fritters at a time. Cook for 3–4 minutes, until the underside of each fritter is golden. Turn over and cook fritters on the other side. Transfer to a plate to keep warm while cooking the remaining fritters in the same way.

4. To serve place two fritters on each plate and top with ¼ cup of roast tomatoes, a small handful of arugula, and finish with a drizzle of olive oil.

Roast Tomatoes

1½ cup cherry tomatoes
4 tablespoons extra-virgin olive oil
sea salt
freshly ground black pepper

1. Preheat the oven to 350°F. Place tomatoes in a skillet or roasting pan in which they fit snugly, and drizzle with olive oil. Sprinkle with sea salt and pepper. Roast in the oven about 20 minutes.

▶ **MODERATE GI**

PER SERVING:

CAL	286
CARB	31 g
FAT	13 g
FIBER	3 g

TABBOULEH

*T*abbouleh is best if you make it ahead, allowing time for the flavors to develop. It keeps a couple of days in the refrigerator. A COOK'S NOTE: Variations include the addition of a chopped cucumber, a crushed clove of garlic, or 2 tablespoons of chopped fresh mint. You can use half lemon juice and half vinegar if preferred.

PREPARATION TIME: 15 minutes ■ **COOKING TIME:** 30 minutes ■ **SERVES** 4

½ cup cracked wheat (bulgur)

1 cup fresh flat-leafed parsley or continental parsley, finely chopped

1 small onion or 3–4 green onions, finely chopped

1 medium tomato, finely chopped

Dressing

2 tablespoons fresh lemon juice

2 tablespoons olive oil

pinch salt

½ teaspoon freshly ground black pepper

1. Cover the bulgur with hot water and soak for 20–30 minutes to soften. Drain well and roll in a clean, lint-free kitchen towel to squeeze out excess water.
2. Combine the bulgur, parsley, onion, and tomato in a bowl.
3. For the dressing, combine all the ingredients in a screw-top jar; shake well.
4. Add the dressing to the bulgur mixture and toss lightly to combine.

▶ **LOW GI**

PER SERVING:

CAL	160
CARB	15 g
FAT	10 g
FIBER	5 g

ASIAN-STYLE SCRAMBLED TOFU

$\mathcal{T}$ofu is an easy way of using soy. It contains very little carbohydrate, so it doesn't have a GI value.

PREPARATION TIME: 5 minutes ■ **COOKING TIME:** 10 minutes ■ **SERVES 4**

---

1 pound firm tofu, patted dry with paper towel

2 tablespoons olive oil

2 tablespooons sweet chili sauce

2 tablespoons salt-reduced soy sauce

⅓ cup chopped coriander

4 thick slices whole-grain bread

> **▶ LOW GI**
>
> **PER SERVING:**
>
> | | |
> |---|---|
> | CAL | 239 |
> | CARB | 18 g |
> | FAT | 14g |
> | FIBER | 7 g |

1. Crumble the tofu into small pieces. Heat the oil in a large wok over high heat, carefully swirling around to coat the side of the wok.
2. Add the tofu and stir-fry for 3–4 minutes or until heated through. Remove the wok from the heat and toss in sweet chili sauce, soy sauce, and coriander.
3. Toast the bread and serve topped with the scrambled tofu. Garnish with chopped cilantro and parsley.

ASPARAGUS, ARUGULA AND LEMON BARLEY "RISOTTO"

*C*lassic risotto is made with Arborio rice, but this creamy variant, made with lower-GI barley, is an unusual twist—*and* incredibly delicious. It's terrific either paired with a side salad, or it makes a wonderful bed for grilled fish.

PREPARATION TIME: 10 minutes ■ SOAKING TIME: overnight
■ COOKING TIME: 30 minutes ■ SERVES 4

---

1 tablespoon olive oil

1 white onion, finely chopped

2 large garlic cloves, finely chopped

1 cup pearl barley, soaked overnight, drained

½ cup white wine

3 cups hot vegetable stock

Finely grated zest of 1 lemon

1 bunch asparagus, trimmed, sliced diagonally

1 bunch arugula, trimmed, leaves shredded

¼ cup lemon juice

⅓ cup finely grated Parmesan

▶ **LOW GI**

PER SERVING:

CAL	337
CARB	47 g
FAT	8g
FIBER	11 g

1. Heat the olive oil in a large heavy-based pan over medium-low heat. Add the onion and cook stirring occasionally for 5 minutes or until soft. Add the garlic and cook, stirring, for 30 seconds longer.

2. Increase the heat to medium, add the barley, and cook, stirring, until the barley is evenly coated in the oil. Add the white wine and let it bubble until reduced by half.

3. Add the lemon zest and start adding the stock a ladleful at a time. Cook, stirring, until almost all the stock has evaporated before adding more stock.

4. When you have added all the stock and the barley is almost tender (this will take about 15–20 minutes), add the asparagus and cook for 3–4 minutes.

5. Remove the risotto from the heat, add the arugula, lemon juice, and Parmesan. Cover and let stand for 3–4 minutes.

WHOLE-WHEAT PENNE WITH ARUGULA AND EDAMAME

*L*ike traditional pasta made from durum wheat, whole-wheat pasta is also low-GI and a higher-fiber choice. Most supermarkets and specialty grocers now carry a variety of sizes and shapes of whole-wheat pasta, alongside the durum choices, so be creative, and enjoy!

PREPARATION TIME: 15 minutes ■ COOKING TIME: 20 minutes ■ SERVES 4

---

2 cups shelled edamame

8 ounces whole-wheat penne

1 tablespoon extra-virgin olive oil, divided

2 cloves garlic, minced

4 cups coarsely chopped arugula

½ cup freshly grated Parmigiano-Reggiano cheese

▶ LOW GI

PER SERVING:

CAL	435
CARB	52 g
FAT	16 g
FIBER	7 g

1. Cook the edamame in boiling salted water until they are crispy but tender. Remove them to a bowl with a slotted spoon.

2. Add the pasta to the same water, and cook according to package directions. Drain it in a colander, drizzle with ½ teaspoon of the oil, and set it aside.

3. In a large nonstick skillet, heat the remaining oil over medium-high heat. Add the garlic and cook 15 seconds. Mix in the arugula, coating it with the oil, and cook until wilted, 2 minutes. Mix in the edamame and remove the pan from the heat. Add the drained pasta, stirring until it is warmed through, and season to taste with salt and pepper.

4. Divide the pasta and vegetables among 4 bowls and top with equal amounts of cheese.

SPICY NOODLES

*G*ood-tasting and good for you, too. Serve as a side dish, or add strips of stir-fried chicken or meat with a package of Asian-style mixed vegetables for a complete meal.

PREPARATION TIME: 10 minutes ■ **COOKING TIME: 15 minutes** ■ **SERVES 4**

---

8 oz dried thin egg noodles

2 teaspoons oil

2 cloves garlic, crushed, or 2 teaspoons minced garlic

1 teaspoon minced ginger

1 teaspoon minced hot peppers

6 green onions, sliced

1 tablespoon smooth peanut butter

2 tablespoons soy sauce

1 cup prepared chicken stock

▶ LOW GI

PER SERVING:

CAL	280
CARB	45 g
FAT	6 g
FIBER	4 g

1. Add the noodles to a large saucepan of boiling water and boil, uncovered, for about 5 minutes or until just tender.
2. While the noodles are cooking, heat the oil in a nonstick frying pan, add the garlic, ginger, hot peppers, and onions and stir-fry for 1 minute. Remove from the heat.
3. Stir in the peanut butter and soy sauce and gradually add the stock, stirring until smooth. Stir over heat until simmering, and simmer for 2 minutes.
4. Drain the noodles and add to the spicy sauce, stirring to coat. Serve immediately.

PASTA WITH
TANGY TOMATOES

A simple, light pasta dish that can be on the plate in about 15 minutes.

PREPARATION TIME: 15 minutes ■ **COOKING TIME:** 15 minutes ■ **SERVES 2**

---

5 oz uncooked spaghetti or other pasta

3 medium tomatoes

1 tablespoon olive oil

1 tablespoon capers, drained

1 clove garlic, crushed, or 1 tablespoon minced garlic

juice of 1 lemon

1 tablespoon hot sauce

black pepper

fresh basil leaves, shredded

1. Cook the spaghetti according to package directions.
2. Meanwhile, dice the tomatoes. Combine in a bowl with the olive oil, capers, garlic, lemon juice, hot sauce, olives, pepper, and basil.
3. Drain the spaghetti and return to its saucepan. Add the tomato combination to it and stir in. Serve hot or warm.

▶ LOW GI

PER SERVING:

CAL	415
CARB	65 g
FAT	10 g
FIBER	7 g

CHICK NUTS

*T*oasted chickpeas make a terrifically healthy low-GI snack. Spice them up with the flavorings suggested or use your own combinations. All you need is some chickpeas.

PREPARATION TIME: 10 minutes ■ SOAKING TIME: overnight
■ COOKING TIME: 45 minutes ■ MAKES 6 Cups

---

1 1-lb package dry chickpeas

▶ LOW GI

PER ½ CUP:

CAL	320
CARB	45 g
FAT	6 g
FIBER	15 g

1. Soak the chickpeas in water overnight. Next day, drain and pat dry with paper towels.
2. Spread the chickpeas in a single layer over a baking tray. Bake at 350°F for about 45 minutes or until completely crisp. (They will shrink to their original size.)
3. Toss with one of the two flavoring options below while hot, or cool and serve plain.

Chick Devils
1. Sprinkle a mixture of cayenne pepper and salt over the hot chick nuts.

Red Chicks
1. Sprinkle a mixture of paprika and garlic salt over the hot chick nuts.
2. After seasoning these, allow them to air dry for a few days to ensure all residual moisture has evaporated.

Main Dishes

■

Vegetable Lasagna

Spinach Pasta with Broccoli Rabe and Scallops

Moroccan Chicken over Couscous

Steamed Mussels over Ratatouille and Basmati Rice

Spicy Beef Stew

Fish Fillets over Sweet Potato Wedges with Oven-Roasted Basil
Tomatoes

Pork and Noodle Stir-fry with Cashews

Glazed Chicken with Sweet Potato Mash and Stir-Fried Greens

Warm Lamb and Chickpea Salad

Spicy Pilaf with Chickpeas

Moroccan Kebabs

Winter Vegetarian Stew

VEGETABLE LASAGNA

Soft layers of spinach, cheese, and lasagna noodles with a luscious vegetable sauce—this is a fabulous all-in-one pan meal that's perfect for a cool evening repast. Dipping the lasagna sheets briefly in hot water before use helps to soften them prior to cooking.

PREPARATION TIME: 35 minutes ■ COOKING TIME: 1 hour 30 minutes ■ SERVES 6

---

1 bunch spinach, washed and stalks removed

8 oz instant lasagna sheets

2 tablespoons grated Parmesan cheese or low-fat cheddar cheese

Vegetable Sauce

2 teaspoons oil

1 medium onion, chopped

2 cloves garlic, crushed, or 2 teaspoons minced garlic

8 oz mushrooms, sliced

1 small green pepper, chopped

1 6-ounce can tomato paste

1 1-lb can beans, any variety, rinsed and drained

1 15-ounce can tomatoes, undrained and mashed

1 teaspoon mixed herbs

Cheese Sauce

1½ tablespoons poly-or monounsaturated margarine

1 tablespoon white flour

1½ cups low-fat milk

½ cup grated low-fat cheese

pinch ground nutmeg

freshly ground black pepper

1. Blanch or lightly steam the spinach until just wilted; drain well.

2. For the vegetable sauce, heat the oil in a nonstick frying pan. Add the onions and garlic and cook for about 5 minutes or until soft. Add the mushrooms and pepper and cook another 3 minutes, stirring occasionally. Add the tomato paste, beans, tomatoes, and herbs. Bring to a boil and simmer, partly covered, for 15 to 20 minutes.

3. Meanwhile, for the cheese sauce, melt the margarine in a saucepan or a microwave bowl. Stir in the flour and cook 1 minute, stirring (for 30 seconds on high, in microwave).

4. Remove from the heat. Gradually add the milk, stirring until smooth. Stir over medium heat until the sauce boils and thickens, or in microwave on high until boiling, stirring occasionally. Remove from heat, stir in the cheese, nutmeg, and pepper.

5. To assemble, pour half the vegetable sauce over the base of a lasagna pan (about 6½ × 10½ inches). Cover with a layer of lasagna sheets, then half the spinach. Spread a thin layer of cheese sauce over the spinach. Top

with the remaining vegetable sauce and remaining spinach. Place over a layer of lasagna sheets and finish with the remaining cheese sauce. Sprinkle with Parmesan or cheddar cheese.

6. Cover with aluminum foil and bake in a moderate oven (350°F) for 40 minutes. Remove foil and bake for a further 30 minutes or until the top is beginning to brown.

▶ LOW GI	
PER SERVING:	
CAL	340
CARB	44 g
FAT	10 g
FIBER	9 g

SPINACH PASTA
WITH BROCCOLI RABE AND SCALLOPS

*T*his is a beautifully balanced and easy-to-prepare low-GI pasta dish—a delicious and not-too-time-consuming midweek meal. Blanching the broccoli rabe in the pasta water reduces its bitterness; the bite of this Italian vegetable is a perfect foil for the earthy mushrooms and the buttery scallops.

PREPARATION TIME: 15 minutes ■ COOKING TIME: 30 minutes ■ SERVES 4

---

1 lb broccoli rabe

salt

8 oz uncooked spinach rotini or penne

1 tablespoon olive oil

2 medium yellow onions, finely diced

3 cloves garlic, crushed, or 1½ tablespoons minced garlic

1 lb shiitake or cremini mushrooms

1 pound fresh scallops

red pepper flakes, to taste

freshly ground black pepper and salt, to taste

¼ cup freshly grated Parmesan cheese

¼ cup chopped fresh parsley

▶ LOW GI

PER SERVING:

CAL	551
CARB	65 g
FAT	8 g
FIBER	4 g

1. Bring a large pot of water to a boil. Meanwhile, discard the lower stems of the broccoli rabe and chop into roughly 3-inch pieces. Wash and drain thoroughly then cook for 2–3 minutes in the boiling, salted water. Remove from the water with tongs, saving the water for the pasta. Immediately plunge the broccoli rabe into ice-cold water, then drain and set aside.

2. Add the pasta to a large pot of boiling water and boil, uncovered, until just tender. Drain and keep warm, reserving ½ cup of the pasta water.

3. While the pasta is cooking, begin the sauce. Heat the oil in a nonstick frying pan. Add the onions, garlic, and mushrooms, and cook for about 5 minutes, until softened. Add the broccoli rabe and cook for about 5 minutes, then add the scallops, and cook for about 5 more minutes, until cooked through.

4. Season with red pepper flakes, to taste, and freshly ground black pepper and salt.

5. Combine the sauce with the pasta, adding reserved pasta water to thin the sauce.

6. Sprinkle with the Parmesan and chopped parsley. Serve hot.

MOROCCAN CHICKEN
OVER COUSCOUS

A dish that is even better the day after, so don't be deterred if you only have a few mouths to feed; you'll all appreciate the leftovers.

PREPARATION TIME: 15 minutes ■ **COOKING TIME:** 20 minutes ■ **SERVES 6**

---

2 teaspoons ground cumin

2 teaspoons ground coriander

1 teaspoon ground fennel

1 15-ounce can chickpeas, drained and patted dry

2 cloves garlic, finely chopped

2 hot red peppers, finely chopped

1 tablespoon olive oil

1 lb chicken-breast cutlets, skinless

½ bunch flat-leafed parsley, coarsely chopped

1 lemon, thinly sliced

½ cup dry white wine

1 cup couscous, uncooked

½ cup raisins

juice of 1 lemon

salt

freshly ground black pepper

▶ MODERATE GI

PER SERVING:

CAL	360
CARB	43 g
FAT	9 g
FIBER	4 g

1. Combine the cumin, coriander, and fennel in a mixing bowl, and toss the chickpeas in the spices.
2. Heat the olive oil in a large wok or frying pan. Add the garlic and hot peppers and cook, stirring, for 1 minute.
3. Toss the chickpeas into the pan and cook until the aroma of the spices comes through—approximately 2 minutes. Place chickpeas in a large bowl and set aside.
4. Add 1 tablespoon olive oil to the pan and cook the chicken cutlets for approximately 4 minutes or until just cooked through. Add to the chickpeas, and stir in the chopped parsley and lemon slices.
5. To make a sauce, deglaze the pan with the wine, simmering for 2 minutes.
6. Pour over the chicken mixture and keep warm.
7. Place the couscous in a large mixing bowl and pour 1 cup of boiling water over the top.
8. As the couscous plumps up, gently mix in the raisins, lemon juice, and salt and pepper.

STEAMED MUSSELS OVER RATATOUILLE AND BASMATI RICE

The ratatouille flavor improves with time, so make it the day before and reheat gently. If you prefer a slightly different taste, try using clams instead of the mussels.

PREPARATION TIME: 45 minutes ■ **COOKING TIME: 1 hour** ■ **SERVES 4**

---

1 large eggplant, cut into small cubes

1 large red pepper, halved, seeded and diced (½-inch pieces)

4 zucchini, sliced into 1-inch rings

1 large onion, roughly chopped

3 cloves garlic, roughly chopped

1 tablespoon mustard seed oil

1 15-ounce can chopped tomatoes, undrained

2 cups water

4 bay leaves

2 sprigs fresh thyme

salt

freshly ground black pepper

8 leaves fresh basil

1 cup basmati rice

1 lb mussels (approximately 20)

1 cup water

2 bay leaves

10 black peppercorns

> ▶ **MODERATE GI**
>
> **PER SERVING:**
>
> | | |
> |---|---|
> | CAL | 390 |
> | CARB | 56 g |
> | FAT | 7 g |
> | FIBER | 6 g |

1. Place the eggplant in a colander, sprinkle with salt, and leave for 30 minutes. Wash under cold water, drain, and pat dry with a paper towel.
2. Heat the oil in a large saucepan and add the eggplant, pepper, zucchini, onion, and garlic. Toss in the hot oil for 2 minutes, then add the tomatoes, water, and herbs. Season with salt and pepper. Reduce the heat and simmer for 45 minutes, stirring occasionally.
3. Remove the bay leaves and thyme sprigs. Chop the basil leaves and stir through the ratatouille.
4. Bring 2 quarts of salted water to a boil and cook the rice for 11 minutes. Immediately drain and keep warm.
5. Prepare the mussels by discarding any broken shells and soaking in cold water. Pull the "beard" from the side of the shell with a sharp tug toward the pointed end of the mussel.
6. Bring the wine and water, bay leaves, and peppercorns to a boil, reduce the heat, and add the mussels. Cover the saucepan with the lid, and simmer for approximately 2 minutes, removing each mussel as it fully opens. Discard any unopened shells.
7. To serve, arrange half a cup of rice in the middle of the plate, top with spoonfuls of ratatouille, and arrange the cooked mussel shells over the top.

SPICY BEEF STEW

*H*ere's a warm comfort food, full of flavor and packed with nutrients.

PREPARATION TIME: 25 minutes ■ **COOKING TIME:** 1 hour 40 minutes ■ **SERVES 8**

---

1 lb rump steak, diced

⅓ cup white flour

salt

freshly ground black pepper

1 tablespoon olive oil

2 medium onions, finely diced

3 cloves garlic, coarsely chopped

1 red hot pepper, coarsely chopped

3 large (3½ lbs) sweet potatoes, peeled and coarsely diced

1½ quarts beef stock

2 tablespoons tomato paste

1 tablespoon grainy mustard

2 stalks celery, sliced

2 large red peppers, halved, seeded, and coarsely diced

1 cup corn kernels

1 28-ounce can peeled chopped tomatoes, undrained

1 15-ounce can pinto beans, drained

1 cup spiral noodles, cooked

½ cup kalamata olives

½ bunch parsley, coarsely chopped

1. Toss the steak in flour seasoned with salt and black pepper in a large mixing bowl.

2. Heat the oil in a large 6-quart casserole dish or metal pan and gently cook the onions, garlic, and hot pepper for 1 minute. Add the steak and brown on all sides.

3. Add the sweet potato, beef stock, tomato paste, grainy mustard, celery, pepper, corn kernels, and tomatoes. Season with salt and pepper. Simmer gently, with lid on, for 1½ hours, stirring occasionally.

4. Remove the lid and add the pinto beans, noodles, and olives. Simmer for 5 minutes, stir in the parsley, and serve immediately.

▶ **LOW GI**

PER SERVING:

CAL	320
CARB	40 g
FAT	7 g
FIBER	8 g

FISH FILLETS OVER
SWEET POTATO WEDGES WITH
OVEN-ROASTED BASIL TOMATOES

$\mathcal{E}$veryone will love the delicate combination of flavors in this dish.

PREPARATION TIME: 20 minutes ■ COOKING TIME: 45 minutes ■ SERVES 6

---

6 large ripe plum tomatoes, halved lengthwise

1 teaspoon olive oil

2 cloves garlic, finely chopped

6 basil leaves, finely sliced

salt

freshly ground pepper

6 small (1½ lbs) fish fillets, such as flounder or halibut

⅓ cup white flour, seasoned with salt and freshly ground black pepper

2 omega-3-enriched eggs, lightly whisked

3 large (1¾ lbs) sweet potatoes, peeled and thinly sliced

2 tablespoons olive oil

3 cups baby spinach leaves

1 tablespoon toasted sesame seeds

6 lemon wedges

▶ LOW GI

PER SERVING:

CAL	310
CARB	26 g
FAT	11 g
FIBER	4 g

1. Preheat the oven to 350°F.

2. Place the tomatoes, cut side up, on a lightly oiled baking tray. Top the tomatoes with a little olive oil, half the garlic, and the basil leaves and seasonings. Place in the oven and bake for 30 minutes.

3. Dip the fish fillets in the seasoned flour and eggs. Cover and set aside in the refrigerator.

4. Peel the sweet potato and slice thinly.

5. Heat 1½ tablespoons olive oil in a heavy-based frying pan and spread the sweet potato slices over it, seasoning the layers with salt and pepper and the remaining garlic. Cook until the underside turns golden brown and slightly crisp, then turn once and cook the other side. Keep warm.

6. Heat ½ tablespoon olive oil in a heavy-based frying pan and cook the fish fillets for approximately 4 minutes, turning once only, until golden brown and flaky.

7. Serve with a bed of baby spinach, and then the sweet potato chips topped with the fish. Sprinkle with toasted sesame seeds and serve with lemon wedges and oven-roasted basil tomatoes.

PORK AND NOODLE STIR-FRY WITH CASHEWS

A classic, flavorful dish that is easy to prepare.

PREPARATION TIME: 20 minutes ■ **COOKING TIME:** 25 minutes ■ **SERVES** 4

---

1 tablespoon oil

1 lb pork strips

10 oz Chinese plain noodles

1 medium red pepper, sliced into thin strips

8 oz broccoli, chopped into small florets

1 clove garlic, crushed

2 teaspoons finely grated fresh ginger

5 oz snow peas, ends cut off and sliced diagonally into thirds

8 oz button mushrooms, thinly sliced

1 baby bok choy, washed, trimmed, and cut lengthways into 8

6 green onions, chopped diagonally

1 tablespoon reduced-sodium soy sauce

1 tablespoon hoisin sauce

1 tablespoon honey

½ cup roasted cashew nuts

▶ LOW GI

PER SERVING:

CAL	580
CARB	56 g
FAT	19 g
FIBER	8 g

1. Heat a large frying pan or wok over high heat. Add half the oil and when the oil is hot, add one-third of the pork strips and stir-fry for 1–2 minutes until just cooked. Repeat with the remaining 2 batches of pork, transferring to a plate covered loosely with foil to keep warm.

2. Prepare the noodles according to package directions and drain.

3. Add the remaining oil to the pan over high heat. Add the pepper, broccoli, garlic, and ginger and stir-fry for about 1 minute. Add the remaining vegetables and stir-fry 1–2 minutes until the vegetables are tender-crisp, sprinkling in a little water if necessary.

4. Combine the sauces and honey together in a bowl.

5. Return the pork to the pan with the noodles and sauces. Toss until well combined and heated through. Put into bowls to serve, and sprinkle with the cashew nuts.

GLAZED CHICKEN WITH SWEET POTATO MASH AND STIR-FRIED GREENS

*H*ere's a yummy stir-fry that's ready in no time.

PREPARATION TIME: 20 minutes ■ COOKING TIME: 35 minutes ■ SERVES 2

Sweet Potato Mash

1 medium sweet potato (1 lb), peeled and cut into chunks

⅓ cup low-fat milk

1 tablespoon sweet chili sauce

Glazed Chicken

2 12-oz chicken breasts, sliced into strips across the grain

1 teaspoon oil

1 cup chicken stock

2 teaspoons reduced-sodium soy sauce

1 tablespoon duck sauce

1 tablespoon cornstarch

2 teaspoons grated fresh ginger

few sprigs of fresh coriander leaves

Stir-fried Greens

1 teaspoon oil

large handful of snow peas

bunch of Chinese greens, such as baby bok choy

2 medium zucchini

1. Boil or microwave the sweet potato until tender. When cooked, drain and mash with milk and sweet chili sauce. Keep warm.

2. Heat a wok or large frying pan with the oil and stir-fry the chicken until browned.

3. Remove from pan and set aside to keep warm.

4. Heat another teaspoon of oil in the wok or frying pan. When hot, add the green vegetables (chopped stalks and sliced zucchini first). Stir-fry until lightly cooked.

5. Combine remaining ingredients in a separate bowl and add to the pan with the cooked chicken and stir until thickened slightly.

6. Serve the chicken and greens over the sweet potato mash.

▶ **LOW GI**

PER SERVING:

CAL	530
CARB	49 g
FAT	15 g
FIBER	9 g

WARM LAMB AND CHICKPEA SALAD

A delicious new way to prepare lamb.

PREPARATION TIME: 20 minutes ■ COOKING TIME: 20 minutes ■ SERVES 4

---

1 lb lamb cutlets

1 tablespoon olive oil

1 onion, finely chopped

3 garlic cloves, crushed

½ teaspoon ground cumin

½ teaspoon ground coriander

½ teaspoon ground ginger

½ teaspoon paprika

2 15-ounce cans chickpeas, drained and rinsed

salt and black pepper to taste

1 tomato, diced

1 cup fresh coriander, finely chopped

1 cup fresh flat-leafed parsley, finely chopped

1 cup fresh mint, finely chopped

3 tablespoons extra-virgin olive oil

juice of 1 lemon

baby spinach leaves, washed, to serve

1. Cook the lamb cutlets in a lightly oiled frying pan, over medium heat, about 3 minutes each side. Transfer to a plate and cover with foil to keep warm. Set aside.

2. Heat the tablespoon of olive oil in the frying pan and cook the onion for 5 minutes or until soft. Add the garlic and spices and cook for 5 minutes over low heat, stirring occasionally. Add the chickpeas and heat through, stirring until warm and well coated with the spice mixture. Remove from the heat and add the salt and pepper, tomato, chopped herbs, extra oil, and lemon juice.

3. Cut the lamb cutlets into thick slices, diagonally. Toss in the chickpea/herb mixture.

4. Arrange the baby spinach leaves on plates and top with the chickpeas and lamb. Serve immediately.

> **▶ LOW GI**
>
> PER SERVING:
>
> | | |
> |---|---|
> | CAL | 430 |
> | CARB | 23 g |
> | FAT | 25 g |
> | FIBER | 9 g |

SPICY PILAF WITH CHICKPEAS

A meatless rice dish that serves 3 to 4 people for a light meal. Two COOK'S NOTES: Garam masala, the key spice here, is a blend of Indian spices (peppercorns, cardamom, cinnamon, cloves, coriander, nutmeg, turmeric, and/or fennel seeds), found in Indian specialty shops, markets, or international sections of large supermarkets. And slivered almonds can be toasted easily by placing in a dry pan over medium heat. Once the pan gets hot, toss the almonds around to toast them. This will take no more than a minute. Don't leave unattended, as the almonds toast rapidly.

PREPARATION TIME: 15 minutes ■ **COOKING TIME:** 20 minutes ■ **SERVES** 3 to 4

---

1 teaspoon poly- or mono-unsaturated margarine

2 teaspoons olive oil

1 medium onion, peeled and finely diced

6 oz button mushrooms, quartered or halved

1 clove garlic, crushed

⅔ cup basmati rice

1 teaspoon garam masala

⅓ 15-ounce can chickpeas, drained

1 bay leaf

1½ cups chicken stock

1 tablespoon slivered almonds, toasted

▶ LOW GI

PER SERVING:

CAL	230
CARB	32 g
FAT	8 g
FIBER	4 g

1. Heat margarine and oil in a medium-sized frying pan over medium heat. Add the onion, cover, and cook 3 minutes, stirring occasionally. Add mushrooms and garlic and cook, uncovered, another 5 minutes, stirring occasionally.

2. Add the rice and spice, stirring to combine until aromatic. Add the chickpeas and bay leaf and pour over stock. Bring to a boil. Reduce heat to very low. Cover with a tight-fitting lid and simmer (without lifting the lid) for at least 12 minutes or until rice is tender and all liquid has been absorbed.

3. Sprinkle with toasted almonds and serve with a salad.

MOROCCAN KEBABS

*H*ere are some North African flavors right from your own kitchen in 20 minutes. Two COOK'S NOTES: Moroccan seasoning is available in jars in the spice section of the supermarket. Alternatively, flavor the patties with 1 clove of crushed garlic and ½ teaspoon each of ground coriander, cumin, paprika, black pepper, and dried rosemary. The optional hummus can be purchased in the refrigerated section of the supermarket or in delicatessens—or make your own using our quick recipe on page 206.

PREPARATION TIME: 15 minutes ■ **COOKING TIME:** 20 minutes ■ **SERVES 4**

---

4 large pieces of pita bread

12 oz lean ground beef

½ cup cracked wheat (bulgur)

2 teaspoons Moroccan seasoning

1 medium white onion, very finely chopped

1 egg, lightly beaten

3 medium tomatoes, diced

1 tablespoon mint, roughly chopped

2 teaspoons olive oil

2 teaspoons red-wine vinegar

lettuce

hummus (optional)

1. Wrap the pita bread in foil and heat in the oven for 15 minutes.
2. Meanwhile, combine beef, bulgur, seasoning, onion, and egg in a bowl. Shape mixture into 8 patties.
3. Heat a nonstick frying pan with cooking spray over medium heat and cook patties about 4 to 5 minutes each side.
4. Combine tomato and mint with olive oil and vinegar in a bowl and serve with the patties and lettuce on the pita bread. Spread with hummus.

▶ **LOW GI**

PER SERVING:

CAL	470
CARB	65 g
FAT	9 g
FIBER	11 g

WINTER VEGETARIAN STEW

A hearty vegetarian meal that can be prepared in around 30 minutes.

PREPARATION TIME: 15 minutes ■ COOKING TIME: 30 minutes ■ SERVE 4 to 6

---

1 15-ounce can kidney beans, rinsed and drained

5 cups water

1 bay leaf

1 teaspoon oil

1 onion, finely chopped

2 cloves garlic, crushed, or 2 teaspoons minced garlic

2 sticks celery, sliced

2 squash or 2 small zucchini, sliced

8 oz button mushrooms

1 28-ounce can tomatoes, undrained and chopped

1 teaspoon minced hot pepper

2 tablespoons tomato paste

1½ cups prepared vegetable stock

1¼ cups small macaroni pasta

freshly ground black pepper

chopped fresh parsley, to serve

1. Heat the oil in a nonstick frying pan, add the onion and garlic and cook for about 5 minutes or until soft.

2. Add the celery, squash, or zucchini and mushrooms and cook, stirring, for 5 minutes.

3. Stir in the beans, tomatoes, hot pepper, tomato paste, and stock, and bring to a boil.

4. Add the pasta, reduce heat, and simmer for about 20 minutes or until the pasta is tender.

5. Add pepper to taste and serve sprinkled with parsley.

▶ **LOW GI**

PER SERVING:

CAL	260
CARB	47 g
FAT	1.5 g
FIBER	12 g

Desserts
and Sweet Treats

■

Cinnamon Muesli Cookies

Granola Bars

Oat Munchies

Mixed Berry and Cinnamon Compote

Oat Bran and Honey Chocolate Pudding

Apple Cranberry Crisp

Cinnamon Raisin Bread and Butter Pudding

Creamy Rice with Sliced Pears

Apricot, Honey and Coconut Crunch

Fresh Fruit Cheesecake

Winter Fruit Salad

Yogurt Berry Jello

CINNAMON MUESLI COOKIES

Good-tasting and good-for-you cookie treats.

PREPARATION TIME: 10 minutes ■ **COOKING TIME:** 25 minutes
■ **MAKES APPROXIMATELY** 10 Cookies

---

2 tablespoons canola oil

3 tablespoons maple syrup

⅓ cup orange juice

1 cup unsweetened rolled-oat muesli

1 cup unbleached all-purpose flour

1½ teaspoons baking powder

¼ teaspoon salt

1 tablespoon cinnamon

powdered sugar

▶ MODERATE GI

PER COOKIE:

CAL	30
CARB	21 g
FAT	4 g
FIBER	2 g

1. Preheat the oven to 350°F.
2. Line a cookie tray with parchment paper.
3. Measure the oil and maple syrup into a large mixing bowl. Add the orange juice and mix.
4. Add the muesli, flour, and cinnamon and mix to a soft dough.
5. Place spoonfuls of the mixture onto the prepared tray, leaving about 1 inch between each cookie.
6. Bake immediately for 15–20 minutes, until just golden brown. Cool on a wire rack and sprinkle with a little powdered sugar.

GRANOLA BARS

𝒯hese bars have a wholesome texture and make a very sustaining snack.

PREPARATION TIME: 20 minutes ■ **COOKING TIME:** 20 minutes ■ **MAKES** 12 Bars

---

½ cup whole-wheat flour

½ cup unbleached all-purpose flour

1¾ teaspoons baking powder

¼ teaspoon salt

½ teaspoon mixed spice

½ teaspoon ground cinnamon

1½ cups rolled oats

1 cup dried-fruit medley or dried fruit of choice, chopped

¼ cup sunflower seed kernels

½ cup apple juice

¼ cup oil

1 egg, lightly beaten

2 egg whites, lightly beaten

1. Line an 8-by-12-inch baking pan with parchment paper.
2. Sift the flours, baking powder, salt, and spices into a large bowl. Stir in the oats, fruit, and seeds and stir to combine.
3. Add the apple juice, oil, and whole egg; mix well. Gently mix in the egg whites until combined.
4. Press the mixture evenly into the prepared pan and press firmly with the back of a spoon. Mark the surface into 12 bars using a sharp knife.
5. Bake in a hot oven (400°F) for about 15 to 20 minutes or until lightly browned. Cool and cut into bars.

▶ LOW GI

PER SERVING:

CAL	140
CARB	15 g
FAT	8 g
FIBER	3 g

OAT MUNCHIES

*C*runchy cookies that make handy low-GI snacks.

PREPARATION TIME: 15 minutes ■ COOKING TIME: 10 minutes
■ MAKES 16 Cookies

6½ tablespoons poly- or monounsaturated margarine

¼ cup honey

1 egg

½ teaspoon vanilla extract

2½ cups rolled oats

2 tablespoons sunflower seed kernels

¼ cup self-rising flour, sifted

▶ **LOW GI**

PER SERVING:

CAL	140
CARB	17 g
FAT	6 g
FIBER	3 g

1. Melt the margarine and honey in a small saucepan.
2. Whisk the egg and vanilla extract together in a large bowl.
3. Add the margarine mixture, oats, sunflower seed kernels, and flour to the egg mixture; stir until combined.
4. Place small spoonfuls of the mixture onto a lightly greased baking tray, spacing evenly.
5. Bake in a moderately hot oven (375°F) for about 10 minutes or until golden brown. Let stand on tray until firm, then loosen and place on a wire rack to cool.

MIXED BERRY AND CINNAMON COMPOTE

*F*ifteen minutes is all it takes for this scrumptious dessert, which is delicious as a topping on your favorite pudding—it pairs beautifully with Cinnamon and Raisin Bread and Butter Pudding (page 280). A COOK'S NOTE: Before you squeeze the oranges for juice, zest the skin using a zester or vegetable peeler.

PREPARATION TIME: 10 minutes ■ **COOKING TIME:** 15 minutes ■ **SERVES** 6 to 8

¾ cup freshly squeezed orange juice

1 cup sugar

2 cinnamon sticks

zest of 1 orange, finely sliced

4 cups mixed berries (raspberries, blackberries, blueberries, strawberries)

1. Place the orange juice, sugar, cinnamon sticks, and orange zest in a large stainless-steel saucepan, and slowly bring to a boil.
2. Add the mixed berries and simmer gently for 2 minutes, just until the berries warm through and swell.
3. Serve warm or as a topping on your favorite pudding.

▶ LOW GI

PER SERVING:

CAL	145
CARB	36 g
FAT	Negligible
FIBER	2 g

OAT BRAN AND
HONEY CHOCOLATE PUDDING

A homey, healthful dessert that includes Nutella in a costarring role.

PREPARATION TIME: 25 minutes ■ COOKING TIME: 55 minutes ■ SERVES 4

---

1 tablespoon raisins

1 tablespoon rum (optional)

4 slices sourdough bread

2 tablespoons Nutella hazelnut spread

2 eggs, lightly beaten

½ teaspoon ground cinnamon

½ cup sugar

1 cup 1% milk

1 tablespoon pudding mix

▶ LOW GI

PER SERVING:

CAL	340
CARB	55 g
FAT	7 g
FIBER	2 g

1. If you want to plump the raisins with rum, place them in a small bowl with the alcohol and heat in the microwave for 20 seconds or until the fruit is swollen.

2. Spread the Nutella thickly over 2 slices of the bread. Dot with the raisins and sandwich together with the remaining 2 slices of bread. Cut each sandwich into 4 triangular quarters and stand upright in a 1-quart baking dish, squashing together to fit.

3. Combine the beaten eggs with the remaining ingredients by whisking together in a deep bowl. Pour the egg mixture over the sandwiches in the baking dish and let stand for 10 minutes while the bread absorbs the custard.

4. Stand the baking dish into another ovenproof dish and add hot water to the larger dish to come halfway up the sides (hot-water-bath style). Bake for 40 minutes at 400°F until the custard around the bread is set and golden in color.

APPLE CRANBERRY CRISP

*T*his is a variation of Jane Brody's recipe in her now-classic *Jane Brody's Good Food Cookbook*—and a delicious late autumn or early winter low-GI dessert. Tart cranberries and sweet apples virtually melt together beneath the crumb topping.

PREPARATION TIME: 15 minutes ■ **COOKING TIME:** 40 minutes ■ **SERVES 8**

---

3 cups cranberries (1 12-ounce package)

2 large apples, peeled, cored and chopped into cranberry-size pieces

½ cup sugar

2 teaspoons cinnamon

¼ cup all-purpose flour, divided

3 tablespoons packed brown sugar

¾ cup cup rolled oats

½ cup chopped walnuts

3 tablespoons mono-or polyunsaturated margarine, melted

> ▶ **LOW GI**
>
> **PER SERVING:**
>
> | | |
> |---|---|
> | CAL | 267 |
> | CARB | 43 g |
> | FAT | 10 g |
> | FIBER | 5 g |

1. Combine the cranberries, apples, sugar, cinnamon, and 1 tablespoon of flour in a mixing bowl. Transfer the mixture to a 6-cup shallow baking dish sprayed with cooking spray.

2. Combine the remaining flour, brown sugar, oats, and nuts, if desired, in the same mixing bowl (it need not be washed). Stir in the melted butter or margarine, and mix the ingredients well—the mixture will be crumbly. Sprinkle the oat mixture over the fruit mixture.

3. Bake the crisp in a preheated 375°F oven for 40 minutes or until the crisp is lightly browned. Let the crisp stand for 10 minutes before serving.

CINNAMON-RAISIN BREAD-AND-BUTTER PUDDING

*S*erved with a mixed-berry compote, this is an ideal early-autumn dessert.

PREPARATION TIME: 20 minutes ■ COOKING TIME: 1 hour ■ SERVES 6 to 8

2½ cups 1% milk

3 omega-3-enriched eggs

2 tablespoons sugar

1 teaspoon vanilla extract

4 slices cinnamon-raisin bread

1 tablespoon margarine

½ cup raisins, soaked in 2 tablespoons brandy

1 teaspoon ground cinnamon

> ▶ **LOW GI**
>
> **PER SERVING:**
>
> | | |
> |---|---|
> | CAL | 175 |
> | CARB | 25 g |
> | FAT | 4 g |
> | FIBER | 1 g |

1. Preheat the oven to 325°F. Lightly grease a 6-cup (1½-quart) ovenproof dish. Boil 4–6 cups of water.

2. Whisk the milk, eggs, sugar, and vanilla extract in a large mixing bowl.

3. Remove the crusts from the bread and spread generously with the margarine, cutting each slice in half diagonally. Stack the triangles of bread upright across the prepared dish. Scatter the cut slices with the presoaked raisins, and pour over the custard mixture. Gently push the slices down to soak up the custard. Sprinkle with cinnamon.

4. Place a deep baking dish in the oven and position the bread-and-butter pudding dish in the center. Pour the boiling water slowly into the baking dish to come at least three-quarters of the way up the sides of the ovenproof dish.

5. Bake for approximately 1 hour or until the custard is set, puffy, and a light golden brown.

6. Serve with the Mixed Berry Compote (page 277).

CREAMY RICE WITH SLICED PEARS

A rice pudding with a healthy twist.

PREPARATION TIME: 10 minutes ■ **COOKING TIME:** 30 minutes ■ **SERVES 4**

---

2 cups water

1 cup Uncle Ben's converted or basmati rice

¾ cup canned evaporated skim milk

¼ cup firmly packed brown sugar

1 teaspoon vanilla extract

1 16-ounce can pear slices, drained

▶ LOW GI

PER SERVING:

CAL	295
CARB	65 g
FAT	Negligible
FIBER	3 g

1. Bring the water to a boil in a saucepan, add the rice and boil for 15 minutes; drain.

2. Return the rice to the saucepan with the milk. Stir over low heat until all the milk is absorbed. Stir in the sugar and vanilla extract; cool.

3. Using an ice cream scoop, serve scoops of rice with the pear slices fanned out next to it.

APRICOT, HONEY
AND COCONUT CRUNCH

*A*pricots, honey, and yogurt on a coconut-cookie base. A COOK'S NOTE: To toast coconut, cook in a nonstick frying pan over low heat, stirring for 2 minutes or until just golden. Remove from the pan to cool.

PREPARATION TIME: 20 minutes ■ COOKING TIME: 45 minutes ■ SERVES 8

Base

¼ cup dried, shredded coconut, toasted

16 oatmeal cookies, finely crushed

4 tablespoons poly-or monounsaturated margarine, melted

Topping

1 cup dried apricots

½ cup boiling water

2 8-ounce containers low-fat apricot yogurt

¼ cup honey

2 eggs

▶ **LOW GI**

PER SERVING:

CAL	255
CARB	32 g
FAT	12 g
FIBER	2 g

1. Line a 6½ × 10½-inch rectangular baking pan with foil.
2. For the base, combine the ingredients in a bowl and mix well. Press the mixture evenly over the base of the prepared pan.
3. Bake in a 350°F oven for about 10 minutes or until browned. Remove from oven and allow to cool.
4. For the topping, cover the apricots with the boiling water, let stand 30 minutes or until soft. Process in a blender or food processor until smooth. Add the yogurt, honey, and eggs and blend until smooth.
5. Spread the topping mixture over the prepared base. Bake in a 350°F oven for about 30 to 35 minutes or until set.
6. Cool, then refrigerate several hours before serving.

FRESH FRUIT CHEESECAKE

A delicious lower-fat cheesecake that leaves you feeling good after you eat it—not weighed down with fat.

PREPARATION TIME: 20 minutes ■ COOKING TIME: 15 minutes
■ CHILLING TIME: 1 hour ■ SERVES 8

Crust

32 oatmeal cookies, crushed

6½ tablespoons poly-or monounsaturated margarine, melted

Filling

2 teaspoons gelatin

2 tablespoons boiling water

1 8-ounce container low-fat fruit yogurt

1 8-ounce container low-fat pineapple cottage cheese

¼ cup honey

½ teaspoon vanilla extract

1 cup chopped fresh fruit (e.g., apple, orange, cantaloupe, strawberries, pear, grapes)

▶ LOW GI

PER SERVING:

CAL	335
CARB	35 g
FAT	14 g
FIBER	1 g

1. For the crust, combine the cookie crumbs and margarine in a bowl. Press evenly into a 9-inch pie dish. Bake in a 350°F oven for 10 minutes. Cool.

2. For the filling, sprinkle the gelatin over the boiling water in a cup, stand cup in a small pan of simmering water and stir until dissolved; cool slightly.

3. Process the cooled gelatin with the yogurt, cottage cheese, honey, and vanilla extract in a blender or food processor until smooth.

4. Arrange the chopped fruit over the prepared crust and pour over the yogurt mixture.

5. Refrigerate for about 1 hour or until set.

■ Don't use papaya, pineapple, or kiwi fruit, as these tend to prevent gelatin from setting.

WINTER FRUIT SALAD

Oranges, apples, and bananas tend to be available year-round, and this combination is ideal when other fruits are out of season.

PREPARATION TIME: 10 minutes ■ **COOKING TIME:** none
■ **CHILLING TIME:** 1 hour ■ **SERVES** 2

---

1 orange, peeled and separated into segments

1 medium red apple, cut into bite-size cubes

2 teaspoons sugar

1 teaspoon fresh lemon juice

1 small banana

1 tablespoon shredded coconut

1. Cut orange segments in half. Place apple and orange chunks in a bowl. Sprinkle with the sugar and lemon juice and mix thoroughly. Cover and refrigerate at least 1 hour.
2. Just before serving, stir in the sliced banana. Sprinkle with coconut to serve.

> ▶ **LOW GI**
>
> **PER SERVING:**
>
> CAL   150
>
> CARB   33 g
>
> FAT   1 g
>
> FIBER   5 g

YOGURT BERRY JELLO

*A*n easy dessert. You could make it with sugar-free gelatin if you wanted to reduce the calories.

PREPARATION TIME: 10 minutes ■ **COOKING TIME:** 5 minutes
■ **CHILLING TIME:** 40 minutes ■ **SERVES 4**

---

1 3-ounce package berry-flavored gelatin powder

1 cup boiling water

1 cup strawberries or frozen raspberries

1½ cups low-fat berry yogurt

▶ LOW GI

PER SERVING:

CAL	85
CARB	16 g
FAT	0 g
FIBER	1 g

1. Stir boiling water into gelatin in a bowl, stir until completely dissolved; cool, but do not allow to set.

2. Roughly chop the strawberries (frozen raspberries will tend to break up on stirring).

3. Fold the yogurt and berries into the gelatin; mix well. Pour into serving dishes, cover, and refrigerate until set.

PART 5

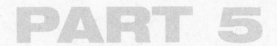

The Authoritative Table of GI Values

■ An Introduction and How to Use the Tables ■

For this all-new third edition of our authoritative table of GI values, we have changed the presentation of our earlier tables considerably—in part because the number of foods tested continues to expand, and in part because we have received many suggestions from readers of the previous editions of this book about its organization. We now present one table, organized alphabetically by category.

These tables will help you put those low-GI food choices into your shopping cart and onto your plate.

Each entry lists an individual food and its GI value. We also list the nominal serving size, the amount of carbohydrate per serving, the GL, and whether the food's GI is low, medium, or high.

High, Medium, or Low GI . . .

- ■ A high GI value is 70 or more.
- ■ A medium/moderate GI value is 56–69 inclusive.
- ■ A low GI value is 55 or less.

You can use the tables to:

▶ find the GI of your favorite foods
▶ compare carb-rich foods within a category (two types of bread or breakfast cereal, for example)

- identify the best carbohydrate choices
- improve your diet by finding a low-GI substitute for high-GI foods
- put together a low-GI meal
- find foods with a high GI but low GL

Each individual food appears alphabetically within a food category, such as "Bread" or "Fruit." This makes it easy to compare the kinds of foods you eat every day and helps you see which high-GI foods you can replace with low-GI versions.

The food categories are listed alphabetically, but if you need to find one quickly, check the category index below. For instance, if you wanted to find the GI value of an apple, you would look under the food category "Fruit."

The food categories used in the tables and the pages on which they begin, are:

- **Beans and legumes**, including baked beans, chickpeas, lentils, and split peas—page **292**
- **Beverages**, including fruit and vegetable juices, soft drinks, flavored milk, and sports drinks—page **293**
- **Bread**, including sliced white and whole-grain bread, fruit breads, flat breads, and crispbreads—page **295**
- **Breakfast cereals**, including processed cereals, muesli, oats, and oatmeal—page **296**
- **Cakes and muffins**, including other baked goods—page **297**
- **Cereal grains**, including couscous, bulgur, and barley—page **298**
- **Cookies and crackers**—page **298**
- **Dairy products**, including milk, yogurt, ice cream, and dairy desserts—page **299**
- **Fruit**, including fresh, canned, and dried fruit—page **301**
- **Gluten-free products**—page **303**
- **Meals**, prepared/convenience—page **303**
- **Meat, seafood and protein**—page **305**
- **Pasta and noodles**—page **306**
- **Rice**—page **307**

- **Snack foods**, including chocolate, fruit bars, muesli bars, nuts and seeds—page **308**
- **Soups**—page **309**
- **Soy products**, including soy milk and soy yogurt—page **311**
- **Spreads and sweeteners**, including sugars, honey, and jam—page **311**
- **Vegetables**, including green vegetables, salad vegetables, and root vegetables—page **312**

In the tables you will sometimes see these symbols:

★ indicates that a food contains little or no carbohydrate. We have included these foods—like vegetables and protein-rich foods—because so many people ask us for their GI.

■ indicates that a food is high in saturated fat. Not all low-GI foods are a good choice; some are too high in saturated fat and sodium for everyday eating. Remember to consider the overall nutritional value of a food.

ⓖ indicates that a food is part of the GI symbol program. Foods with the GI symbol have had their GI tested properly and are a healthy choice for their food category.

To make a fair comparison, all foods have been tested using an internationally standardized method. Gram for gram of carbohydrates, the higher the GI, the higher the blood glucose levels after consumption. If you can't find the GI value in these tables for a food you eat regularly, check out our Web site (www.glycemicindex.com), where we maintain an international database of published GI values that have been tested by a reliable laboratory. Alternatively, please write to the manufacturer and encourage them to have the food tested by an accredited laboratory. In the meantime, choose a similar food from the tables as a substitute.

The GI values in this book are correct at the time of publication. However, the formulation of commercial foods can change and the GI may change as well. You can rely on foods showing the GI symbol. Although some manufacturers include the GI on the nutritional label, you would need to know that the testing was carried out independently by an accredited laboratory.

BEANS & LEGUMES

Food	GI Value	Nominal Serving Size	Available Carbs	GL Value	GI Level
Baked beans, canned in tomato sauce, Heinz®	55	½ cup	17	9	low
Black beans, boiled	30	¾ cup	25	5	low
Black-eyed peas, soaked, boiled	42	¾ cup	29	12	low
Butter beans, dried, boiled	31	½ cup	20	6	low
Butter beans, canned, drained	36	¼ cup	12	4	low
Cannellini beans, canned	31	½ cup	12	4	low
Channa dal (Bengal gram dal)	11	½ cup	11	1	low
Chickpeas, canned	40	½ cup	22	9	low
Chickpeas, dried, boiled	28	¾ cup	24	7	low
Haricot/Navy beans	33	⅔ cup	19.8	7	low
Kidney beans, dark red, canned, drained	43	½ cup	25	7	low
Kidney beans, red, canned, drained	36	½ cup	17	9	low
Kidney beans, red, dried, boiled	28	¾ cup	25	7	low
Kidney beans, red, soaked overnight, boiled	51	¾ cup	24	12	low
Lentils, green, canned	48	½ cup	17	9	low
Lentils, green or brown, dried, boiled	30	¾ cup	17	5	low
Lentils, red, dried, boiled	26	¾ cup	18	5	low
Lima beans, baby, frozen, reheated	32	½ cup	30	10	low
Low-Fat 4-Bean Salad; President's Choice®Blue Menu™	13	⅓ cup	9	1	low
Mung beans	39	½ cup	17	5	low
Refried beans, canned	38	½ cup	20	8	low
Soybeans, canned, drained	14	½ cup	6	1	low
Soybeans, dried, boiled	18	¾ cup	6	1	low
Split peas, yellow, boiled	32	¾ cup	19	6	low
White beans, canned	38	½ cup	31	12	low
White beans, dried, boiled	33	¾ cup	31	10	low

★ little or no carbohydrate   ▮ high in saturated fat   © program participant

BEVERAGES

Food	GI Value	Nominal Serving Size	Available Carbs	GL Value	GI Level
Allsport®, orange	53	8 fl oz	17	9	low
Ⓖ Apple and cherry juice, unsweetened	43	8 fl oz	33	14	low
Ⓖ Apple and mango juice, unsweetened	47	8 fl oz	27	12	low
Apple juice, clear, no added sugar	40	8 fl oz	28	11	low
Ⓖ Apple juice, filtered, no added sugar	44	8 fl oz	30	13	low
Ⓖ Apple juice with fiber	37	8 fl oz	28	10	low
Banana smoothie, soy drink, low-fat	30	8 fl oz	22	7	low
Beer (4.6% alcohol)	66	8 fl oz	10	7	med
Carrot juice, freshly made	43	8 fl oz	23	10	low
Coffee, black, no milk or sugar	★	8 fl oz	0	0	
Cranberry Juice Cocktail, Ocean Spray®	52	8 fl oz	31	16	low
Ensure®, vanilla, nutritional supplement	48	8 fl oz	34	16	low
Fanta®, orange soft drink	68	8 fl oz	34	23	med
Gatorade® sports drink	78	8 fl oz	15	12	high
Grapefruit juice, unsweetened	48	8 fl oz	22	9	low
Malted milk powder in reduced-fat milk	40	8 fl oz	31	12	low
Malted milk powder in skim milk	46	8 fl oz	24	11	low
Malted milk powder in whole milk n	45	8 fl oz	24	11	low
Nestle Quik® powder, chocolate, in reduced-fat milk	41	8 fl oz	11	5	low
Nestle Quik® powder, strawberry, in reduced-fat milk	35	8 fl oz	12	4	low
Orange juice, unsweetened, fresh	50	8 fl oz	18	9	low
Orange juice, unsweetened, from concentrate	53	8 fl oz	18	9	low
Orange Delight Juice Beverage, President's Choice® Blue Menu™	48	8 fl oz	16	8	low
Pineapple juice, unsweetened	46	8 fl oz	34	16	low
POM Wonderful® 100% Pomegranate Juice, no added sugars	67	8 fl oz	40	27	med
POM Wonderful® Pomegranate Blueberry 100% Juice, no added sugars	58	8 fl oz	39	23	med
Prune juice, unsweetened	43	8 fl oz	30	13	low
Rice milk, average	92	8 fl oz	34	31	high
Rice milk, calcium-enriched Vitasoy®	79	8 fl oz	22	17	high
Schweppes Lemonade	54	8 fl oz	28	15	low
Slim-Fast® drink, can, vanilla or chocolate	39	8 fl oz	39	15	low

★ little or no carbohydrate   ■ high in saturated fat   Ⓖ program participant

BEVERAGES

Food	GI Value	Nominal Serving Size	Available Carbs	GL Value	GI Level
Slim-Fast® drink powder, all flavors, made with skim milk	35	8 fl oz	34	12	low
Soda, Coca-Cola®	53	8 fl oz	26	14	low
Soda, diet varieties	★	8 fl oz	0	0	
Soy Beverage, Original, President's Choice® Blue Menu™	15	8 fl oz	9	1	low
Soy Beverage, Chocolate, President's Choice® Blue Menu™	40	8 fl oz	28	11	low
Soy Beverage, Vanilla, President's Choice® Blue Menu™	28	8 fl oz	16	4	low
Soy milk, full fat, calcium-fortified	36	8 fl oz	18	6	low
Soy milk, reduced-fat, calcium-fortified	44	8 fl oz	17	8	low
Tomato Juice, Low Sodium, President's Choice® Blue Menu™	23	8 fl oz	7	2	low
Tomato juice, no added sugar	38	8 fl oz	9	4	low
Trim Advantage® meal replacement shake, Vanilla or Chocolate Mocha, 2 scoops +Quixtar	23	8.5 fl oz	21	5	low

★ little or no carbohydrate   ■ high in saturated fat   Ⓖ program participant

BREAD

Food	GI Value	Nominal Serving Size	Available Carbs	GL Value	GI Level
Ⓖ 9 Grain mutigrain bread	43	1 slice	14	6	low
Bagel, white	72	1 small (2.5 oz)	35	25	high
Chapatti, baisen (India)	27	¼ cup	23.3	6	low
Dinner roll, white	73	1 small (1 oz)	16	12	high
Flaxseed and soy bread	55	1 slice	24	13	low
Gluten-free, multigrain bread	79	1 slice	13	10	high
Hamburger bun, white	61	½ bun (1 oz)	15	9	med
Kaiser roll, white	73	½ roll (1 oz)	16	12	high
Multigrain Flax Loaf, President's Choice® Blue Menu™	51	2 slices	32	16	low
Ⓖ Oat bran and honey bread	45	1 slice	13	7	low
Pita bread, 4", white	57	1 pita	17	10	med
Pumpernickel bread	50	1 slice	10	5	low
Raisin bread	63	1 slice	17	11	med
Rye bread, black	76	1 slice	13	10	high
Rye bread, dark	86	1 slice	14	12	high
Rye bread, light	68	1 slice	14	10	med
Ⓖ Rye bread, seeded	51	1 slice	13	7	low
Sourdough rye bread	48	1 slice	12	6	low
Sourdough wheat bread	54	1 slice	14	8	low
Spelt multigrain bread	54	1 slice	12	7	low
Stuffing, bread	74	½ cup	21	16	high
Sunflower and barley bread	57	1 slice	11	6	med
Taco shells, cornmeal-based, baked	68	2 shells	12	8	med
Tortillas, Whole Wheat, President's Choice® Blue Menu™	59	1 tortilla	27	16	med
Tortillas, Flax, President's Choice® Blue Menu™	53	1 tortilla	29	15	low
White bread, enriched, sliced	71	1 slice	14	10	high
Whole wheat bread, made w/enriched wheat flour, sliced	71	1 slice	12	9	high
Whole wheat bread, 100%, stoneground	59	1 slice	12	7	med
Whole Wheat Soy Loaf, President's Choice® Blue Menu™	45	2 slices	27	12	low
Wonder White®, bread, sliced	80	1 slice	15	12	high

★ little or no carbohydrate   ▪ high in saturated fat   Ⓖ program participant

BREAKFAST CEREALS

Food	GI Value	Nominal Serving Size	Available Carbs	GL Value	GI Level
All-Bran®, Kellogg's®	34	½ cup	15	5	low
Bran Flakes, Kellogg's®	74	¾ cup	18	13	high
Bran Flakes, President's Choice® Blue Menu™	65	¾ cup	19	12	med
Coco Pops®, Kellogg's®	77	1 cup	26	20	high
Corn Flakes®, Kellogg's®	77	1 cup	25	20	high
Corn Pops®, Kellogg's®	80	1 cup	26	21	high
Crispix®	87	1 cup	25	22	high
Fiber First Multi-Bran Cereal, President's Choice® Blue Menu™	56	½ cup	10	6	med
Froot Loops®, Kellogg's®	69	1 cup	26	18	med
Frosted Flakes®, Kellogg's®	55	¾ cup	26	15	low
Granola Clusters, Low Fat, Original, President's Choice® Blue Menu™	63	⅔ cup	40	25	med
Granola Clusters, Low Fat, Raisin & Almond, President's Choice® Blue Menu™	70	⅔ cup	40	28	med
Honey Smacks®, Kellogg's®	71	1 cup	23	16	high
Muesli, natural	40	¼ cup	18	8	low
Muesli, Swiss Formula	56	¼ cup	16	9	low
Muesli, toasted	43	¼ cup	17	7	low
Nutri-Grain®, Kellogg's®	66	½ cup	15	10	med
Oat bran, raw, unprocessed	55	2 Tbsp.	5	3	low
Oatmeal, instant, made with water	82	1 cup	26	17	high
Oatmeal, from old-fashioned oats, made with water	58	1 cup	21	11	med
Oatmeal, from steel-cut oats, made with water	52	1 cup	22	11	low
Puffed buckwheat	65	1 cup	12	8	med
Puffed rice	80	2 cups	21	17	high
Puffed wheat	80	2 cups	21	17	high
Rice bran, unprocessed	19	4 Tbsp.	14	3	low
Raisin Bran®, Kellogg's®	73	½ cup	19	14	high
Rice Krispies®, Kellogg's®	82	1¼ cups	26	22	high
Semolina, wheat, hot cereal, made with water	55	⅔ cup	11	6	low
Shredded Wheat	75	½ cup	20	15	high
Special K®, Kellogg's®	56	1 cup	21	11	med
Weet-Bix, biscuits, regular	69	½ cup	17	12	med

★ little or no carbohydrate   ■ high in saturated fat   Ⓖ program participant

CAKES & MUFFINS

Food	GI Value	Nominal Serving Size	Available Carbs	GL Value	GI Level
Angel food cake, plain ■	67	⅛ cake (2 oz)	29	19	med
Apple muffin, home-made ■	46	1 sm (4 oz)	29	13	low
Banana bread, home-made ■	51	1 slice (3 oz)	38	18	low
Blueberry Bran Muffin, NutriSystem®	28	2 oz	11	3	low
Blueberry muffin, commercially-made ■	59	1 sm (2 oz)	29	17	med
Bran muffin, commercially-made ■	60	1 sm (2 oz)	24	15	med
Carrot muffin, commercially-made ■	62	1 sm (2 oz)	32	20	med
Chocolate cake, cake mix with frosting, Betty Crocker ■	38	½₁₂ cake (3.5 oz)	52	20	low
Chocolate Fudge Cake, NutriSystem®*	25	1.5 oz	16	4	low
Croissant, plain ■	67	1 sm (2 oz)	26	17	med
Crumpet, white	69	1 sm (2 oz)	19	13	med
Cupcake with strawberry icing ■	73	1 sm (1.5 oz)	26	19	high
Pancakes, 6", prepared from pancake mix ■	67	1 pancake	23	15	med
Pound cake, plain, Sara Lee ■	54	1 slice (1.75 oz)	23	12	low
Scones, plain, made from package mix	92	1 oz	9	8	high
Sponge cake, plain, unfilled ■	46	⅛ cake (2 oz)	36	17	low
Vanilla cake, cake mix with vanilla frosting, Betty Crocker ■	42	½₁₂ cake (3.5 oz)	58	24	low
Waffles, plain ■	76	1 oz	13	10	high

*NutriSystem® Nourish™ products are at www.nutrisystem.com

★ little or no carbohydrate   ■ high in saturated fat   Ⓖ program participant

CEREAL GRAINS

Food	GI Value	Nominal Serving Size	Available Carbs	GL Value	GI Level
Buckwheat, boiled	54	¾ cup	30	16	low
Bulgur, cracked wheat, ready to eat	48	½ cup	26	12	low
Couscous, boiled	65	1 cup	33	21	med
Millet, boiled	71	¾ cup	36	25	high
Polenta (cornmeal), cooked with water	68	⅔ cup	13	9	med
Quinoa, boiled	51	¾ cup	17	9	low
Rye berries, boiled	34	¾ cup	38	13	low
Whole-wheat berries, boiled	41	¾ cup	34	14	low

COOKIES & CRACKERS

Food	GI Value	Nominal Serving Size	Available Carbs	GL Value	GI Level
Ancient Grains Snack Crackers, President's Choice® Blue Menu™	65	10 crackers	12	8	med
Arrowroot biscuits	69	1 oz	18	12	med
Breton wheat crackers ■	67	1 oz	14	10	med
Cranberry Orange Cookies, President's Choice® Blue Menu™	60	2 cookies	16	10	med
Crunchy Oat Cookies, President's Choice® Blue Menu™	62	2 cookies	15	9	med
Digestives®, cookies, plain ■	59	1 oz	16	10	med
Gluten-free chocolate-coated cookie	35	1 oz	14	5	low
Ginger & Lemon Cookies, President's Choice® Blue Menu™	64	2 cookies	16	10	med
Graham crackers, plain ■	77	1 oz	18	14	high
Melba toast, plain	70	1 oz	23	16	high

★ little or no carbohydrate   ■ high in saturated fat   Ⓖ program participant

COOKIES & CRACKERS

Food	GI Value	Nominal Serving Size	Available Carbs	GL Value	GI Level
Oatmeal cookies, plain ■	54	2 cookies (1 oz)	17	9	low
Rice cakes, white	82	1 oz	21	17	high
Rich Tea Biscuits® ■	55	1 oz	19	10	low
Ryvita® Country Grains crispbread	65	1 oz	12	8	med
Ryvita® Fruit Crunch crispbread	66	1 oz	20	13	med
Ryvita® Original Rye crispbread	65	1 oz	12	8	med
Ryvita® Sesame Rye crispbread	64	1 oz	12	8	med
Shortbread, plain ■	64	2 cookies (1 oz)	16	10	med
Stoned Wheat Thins®	67	1 oz	17	12	med
Vanilla wafer, 7 small plain ■	77	wafers (1 oz)	18	14	high
Wheat Snack Crackers, President's Choice® Blue Menu™	65	9 crackers	14	9	med
Wheat & Onion Snack Crackers, President's Choice® Blue Menu™	60	9 crackers	14	8	med
Wheat & Sesame Snack Crackers, President's Choice® Blue Menu™	56	9 crackers	14	8	med

DAIRY PRODUCTS

Food	GI Value	Nominal Serving Size	Available Carbs	GL Value	GI Level
Cheese ■	★	1 oz	0	0	
Custard, traditional, home-made ■	43	½ cup	17	7	low
Frozen Yogurt, Mochaccino, President's Choice® Blue Menu™	51	½ cup	21	11	low
Frozen Yogurt, Strawberry Banana, President's Choice® Blue Menu™	55	½ cup	20	11	low
Frozen Yogurt, Vanilla, President's Choice® Blue Menu™	46	½ cup	21	10	low
Gelato, sugar-free, chocolate	37	1 cup	14	5	low
Gelato, sugar-free, vanilla	39	1 cup	14	5	low

★ little or no carbohydrate   ■ high in saturated fat   ⓖ program participant

DAIRY PRODUCTS

Food	GI Value	Nominal Serving Size	Available Carbs	GL Value	GI Level
Ⓖ Ice cream, low-fat, chocolate	49	½ cup	14	7	low
Ⓖ Ice cream, low-fat, vanilla	46	½ cup	6	3	low
Ice cream, full-fat, vanilla ■	47	½ cup	15	8	low
Ice cream, full-fat, chocolate ■	37	½ cup	9	4	low
Milk, 1%, light, low-fat	32	8 fl oz	12	4	low
Milk, 2%, reduced-fat	30	8 fl oz	14	4	low
Milk, fat free, skim, nonfat	32	8 fl oz	12	4	low
Milk, whole, full fat ■	27	8 fl oz	12	4	low
Milk, chocolate, low fat, with aspartame	24	8 fl oz	15	3	low
Milk, chocolate, low fat, with sugar	34	8 fl oz	26	9	low
Milk, condensed milk, sweetened, full fat ■	61	2 fl oz	28	17	med
Yogurt, fat-free, with sugar, French Vanilla	40	3.5 oz	27	10	low
Yogurt, fat-free, with sugar, Mango	39	3.5 oz	25	10	low
Yogurt, fat-free, with sugar, Strawberry	38	3.5 oz	22	8	low
Yogurt, fat-free, with sugar, Wild Berry	38	3.5 oz	22	8	low
Yogurt, fat-free, with sugar, average, various flavors	40	7 oz	31	12	low
Yogurt, low fat, no added sugar, vanilla or fruit	20	7 oz	13	3	low
Yogurt, low fat, with sugar, Apricot, Mango and Peach	26	3.5 oz	15	4	low
Yogurt, low fat, with sugar, French Vanilla	26	3.5 oz	18	5	low
Yogurt, low fat, with sugar, Wild Berry	28	3.5 oz	15	4	low
Yogurt, low fat, with sugar, Strawberry	28	3.5 oz	15	4	low
Yoplait Lite Apricot yogurt	27	7 oz	31	9	low
Yoplait Lite Blueberry yogurt	25	7 oz	34	9	low
Yoplait Lite Creamy Vanilla yogurt	27	7 oz	35	9	low
Yoplait Lite Peach Mango yogurt	37	7 oz	31	12	low
Yoplait Lite Strawberry yogurt	25	7 oz	32	8	low
Yoplait Lite Vanilla Strawberry yogurt	25	7 oz	34	8	low
Yoplait No Fat Black Cherry yogurt	16	7 oz	13	2	low
Yoplait No Fat French Cheesecake yogurt	18	7 oz	14	3	low
Yoplait No Fat French Vanilla yogurt	20	7 oz	13	3	low
Yoplait No Fat Raspberry yogurt	16	7 oz	13	2	low
Yoplait No Fat Strawberry yogurt	16	7 oz	12	2	low
Yoplait No Fat Tropical yogurt	20	7 oz	13	3	low

★ little or no carbohydrate   ■ high in saturated fat   Ⓖ program participant

FRUIT, CANNED

Food	GI Value	Nominal Serving Size	Available Carbs	GL Value	GI Level
Apricots, in light syrup	64	½ cup	19	12	med
Fruit cocktail, in natural juice	55	½ cup	16	9	low
Lychees, in syrup, drained	79	½ cup	20	16	high
Peaches, in heavy syrup	58	½ cup	15	9	med
Peaches, in light syrup	57	½ cup	18	9	med
Peaches, in natural juice	45	½ cup	11	4	low
Pear halves, in light syrup	25	½ cup	14	4	low
Pears, in natural juice	44	½ cup	13	5	low

FRUIT, DRIED

Food	GI Value	Nominal Serving Size	Available Carbs	GL Value	GI Level
Apple	29	2 oz	34	10	low
Apricots	30	2 oz	28	9	low
Cranberries, sweetened	64	1.5 oz	29	19	med
Dates, Arabic, vacuum-packed	39	2 oz	41	16	low
Dates, pitted	45	2 oz	40	18	high
Figs, dried	61	2 oz	26	16	med
Prunes, pitted, Sunsweet®	29	2 oz	33	10	low
Raisins	64	2 oz	44	28	med

★ little or no carbohydrate   ▮ high in saturated fat   Ⓖ program participant

FRUIT, FRESH

Food	GI Value	Nominal Serving Size	Available Carbs	GL Value	GI Level
Apple	38	1 sm (4 oz)	15	6	low
Apricots	57	3 sm (6 oz)	13	7	med
Avocado	★	2 Tbsp.	0	0	
Banana, ripe	52	1 sm (4 oz)	26	13	low
Blueberries, wild	53	½ cup	12	7	low
Cantaloupe	67	½ cup	6	4	med
Cherries, dark	63	1 cup	12	3	med
Custard apple	54	1 sm (4 oz)	19	10	low
Grapefruit	25	½ large	11	3	low
Grapes	53	1 cup	18	8	low
Kiwi fruit	53	1 med (4 oz)	12	6	low
Lemon	★	1 sm	0	0	
Lime	★	1 sm	0	0	
Mango	51	½ med (4 oz)	17	8	low
Orange	42	1 sm (4 oz)	11	5	low
Papaya	56	½ sm (4 oz)	8	5	med
Peach	42	1 med (4 oz)	11	5	low
Pear	38	1 med (4 oz)	11	4	low
Pineapple	59	¾ cup	10	6	med
Plum	39	1 med (4 oz)	12	5	low
Raspberries	★	½ cup	0	0	
Rhubarb	★	1 cup	0	0	
Strawberries	40	1 cup	3	1	low
Watermelon	76	¾ cup	6	4	high

★ little or no carbohydrate ■ high in saturated fat Ⓖ program participant

GLUTEN-FREE PRODUCTS

Food	GI Value	Nominal Serving Size	Available Carbs	GL Value	GI Level
Gluten-free buckwheat pancakes 6", from pancake mix	102	1 pancake	22	22	high
Gluten-free chocolate-coated cookie	35	1 oz	14	5	low
Gluten-free corn pasta, cooked	78	1¼ cups	42	32	high
Gluten-free multigrain bread	79	1 slice	13	10	high
Gluten-free rice and corn pasta, cooked	76	1¼ cups	49	37	high

MEALS, PREPARED & CONVENIENCE

Food	GI Value	Nominal Serving Size	Available Carbs	GL Value	GI Level
Chicken nuggets, frozen, reheated ■	46	3.5 oz	16	7	low
Fish sticks ■	38	3.5 oz	19	7	low
French fries, frozen, reheated ■	75	5 oz	29	22	high
Ⓖ Lean Cuisine®, Burmese Vegetable Curry and Rice	50	5 oz	20	9	low
Ⓖ Lean Cuisine®, Chicken Pomodoro	47	5 oz	18	9	low
Lean Cuisine®, French-style Chicken with Rice	36	14 oz	72	26	low
Ⓖ Lean Cuisine®, Honey Soy Beef	47	5 oz	20	9	low
NutriSystem®, Beef Stroganoff with Noodles	41	9 oz	22	9	low
NutriSystem®, Cheese Tortellini	41	7.6 oz	22	9	low
NutriSystem®, Chicken Cacciatore	27	7.6 oz	16	4	low
NutriSystem®, Chicken Pasta Parmesan	41	9 oz	23	9	low
NutriSystem®, Hearty Beef Stew	39	7.6 oz	15	6	low
NutriSystem®, Lasagna with Meat Sauce	26	8.1 oz	26	7	low
NutriSystem®, Pasta with Beef	30	7.6 oz	18	5	low
NutriSystem®, Pasta with Beef and Cheese	33	2.1 oz	26	9	low
NutriSystem®, Pot Roast	31	10 oz	16	5	low
NutriSystem®, Rotini and Meatballs	29	9 oz	25	7	low

★ little or no carbohydrate   ■ high in saturated fat   Ⓖ program participant

MEALS, PREPARED & CONVENIENCE

Food	GI Value	Nominal Serving Size	Available Carbs	GL Value	GI Level
NutriSystem®, Thin Crust Pizza	36	3.2 oz	15	5	low
NutriSystem®, Whipped Sweet Potatoes	36	1.8 oz	24	9	low
Pizza Hut, Pizza, Super Supreme, pan ■	36	3.5 oz	24	9	low
Pizza Hut, Pizza, Super Supreme, thin and crispy ■	30	3.5 oz	22	7	low
Pizza Hut, Pizza, Vegetarian Supreme, thin and crispy ■	49	7 oz	50	25	low
President's Choice® Blue Menu™ Barley Risotto withHerbed Chicken Entrée	38	1 tray	37	14	low
President's Choice® Blue Menu™ Cauliflower-Topped Shepherd's Pie	21	¼ pie	13	3	low
"President's Choice® Blue Menu™ Chicken Curry with Vegetables Entree	26	1 tray	9	2	low
President's Choice® Blue Menu™ Lentil & Bean Vegetarian Patty, Frozen	55	1 patty	27	15	low
President's Choice® Blue Menu™ Low Fat 4 Bean Salad,	13	⅓ cup	9	1	low
President's Choice® Blue Menu™ Penne with Roasted Vegetables Entrée	39	1 tray	43	17	low
President's Choice® Blue Menu™ 3-Rice Bayou Blend Rice & Beans Side Dish	44	¼ pack	34	16	low
President's Choice® Blue Menu™ 4-Rice Pilaf Rice & Beans Side Dish	46	¼ pack	36	16	low
President's Choice® Blue Menu™ Rice & Lentils Espana Side Dish	49	¼ pack	36	17	low
President's Choice® Blue Menu™ Rotini with Chicken Pesto Entrée	57	1 tray	41	23	med
President's Choice® Blue Menu™ Sesame Ginger Chicken & Vegetables Entree	44	1 tray	16	7	low
President's Choice® Blue Menu™ Tomato & Herb Chicken with Vegetables Entree	29	1 tray	11	3	low
President's Choice® Blue Menu™ Yellow Curry Chicken with Vegetables Entree	25	1 tray	14	3	low
President's Choice® Blue Menu™ 9-Vegetable Vegetarian Patty, Frozen	54	1 patty	25	13	low

★ little or no carbohydrate ■ high in saturated fat Ⓖ program participant

MEAT, SEAFOOD & PROTEIN

Food	GI Value	Nominal Serving Size	Available Carbs	GL Value	GI Level
Bacon, lean ■	★	2 med strips (½ oz)	0	0	
Beef, ground, lean	★	3 oz	0	0	
Beef pot pie, with crust ■	45	3.5 oz	27	12	low
Beef, steak, lean	★	3 oz	0	0	
Calamari rings, squid, plain, without batter or bread crumbs	★	3 oz	0	0	
Chicken, without the skin and bone	★	3 oz	0	0	
Chicken nuggets, with breading, frozen, reheated ■	46	3.5 oz	16	7	low
Clams, plain, steamed	★	3 oz	0	0	
Crabmeat, plain, without breading	★	3 oz	0	0	
Duck, without the skin and bone ■	★	3 oz	0	0	
Fish, all-types, fresh or frozen, without skin	★	3 oz	0	0	
Fish sticks, lightly breaded ■	38	3.5 oz	19	7	low
Ham, lean ■	★	3 oz	0	0	
Lamb, lean	★	3 oz	0	0	
Lobster, plain, cooked	★	3 oz	0	0	
Oysters, plain, raw or cooked	★	3 oz	0	0	
Pork, lean	★	3 oz	0	0	
Salami ■	★	1 oz	0	0	
Salmon, canned in water	★	3 oz	0	0	
Sardines, canned	★	2 oz	0	0	
Scallops, plain, cooked	★	3 oz	0	0	
Shrimp, plain, cooked	★	3 oz	0	0	
Sushi, salmon	48	3.5 oz	36	17	low
Tuna, canned in water	★	3 oz	0	0	
Turkey, without the skin and bone	★	3 oz	0	0	
Veal	★	3 oz	0	0	

★ little or no carbohydrate   ■ high in saturated fat   © program participant

PASTA & NOODLES

Food	GI Value	Nominal Serving Size	Available Carbs	GL Value	GI Level
Capellini, white, boiled	45	1 cup	45	20	low
Cheese tortellini, cooked ■	50	6 oz	21	10	low
Corn pasta, gluten-free, cooked	78	1¼ cups	42	32	high
Fettuccine, egg noodles, cooked	40	1 cup	46	18	low
Fuselli twists, tricolor, boiled	51	½ cup	34	17	low
Gnocchi, cooked	68	6 oz	48	33	med
Instant noodles, 99% fat free, dry, package	67	2.5 oz	51	34	med
Linguine, thick, durum wheat, cooked	46	1 cup	48	22	low
Linguine, thin, durum wheat, cooked	52	1 cup	45	23	low
Macaroni and cheese, Kraft® ■	64	1¼ cups	51	32	med
Macaroni, white, durum wheat, cooked	47	1¼ cups	48	23	low
Macaroni, white, plain, cooked	47	1¼ cups	48	18	low
Mung bean noodles, cooked	33	1¼ cups	45	15	low
Ravioli, meat-filled, durum wheat flour, cooked ■	39	6 oz	38	15	low
Rice and corn pasta, gluten-free	76	1¼ cups	49	37	high
Rice pasta, brown, cooked	92	1 cup	38	35	high
Rice vermicelli, cooked	58	1¼ cups	39	22	med
Soba noodles, instant, served in soup	46	1¼ cups	49	22	low
Spaghetti, protein-enriched, cooked	27	1¼ cups	52	14	low
Spaghetti, white, durum wheat, cooked	44	1 cup	48	21	low
Spaghetti, whole wheat, cooked	42	1¼ cups	42	16	low
Spirali, white, durum wheat, cooked	43	1¼ cups	44	19	low
Star Pastina, white, cooked	38	1 cup	48	18	low
Udon noodles, cooked	62	1¼ cups	48	30	med
Vermicelli, white, durum wheat, cooked	35	1 cup	44	16	low
100% Whole Wheat Spaghetti Pasta, President's Choice® Blue Menu™	45	⅕ pack	56	25	low
100% Whole Wheat Rotini Pasta, President's Choice® Blue Menu™	57	⅕ pack	56	32	med

★ little or no carbohydrate ■ high in saturated fat Ⓖ program participant

RICE

Food	GI Value	Nominal Serving Size	Available Carbs	GL Value	GI Level
Arborio risotto rice, white, boiled	69	¾ cup	43	29	med
Basmati rice, white, boiled	58	1 cup	38	22	med
Brown rice, boiled	66	1 cup	37	24	med
Glutinous rice, white, cooked	98	¾ cup	32	31	high
Instant rice, white, boiled	87	¾ cup	42	29	high
Jasmine rice, white, long-grain, cooked	109	¾ cup	42	46	high
Long-grain rice, white, boiled	50	¾ cup	41	23	low
3-Rice Bayou Blend Rice & Beans Side Dish, President's Choice® Blue Menu™	44	¼ pack	34	16	low
4-Rice Pilaf Rice & Beans Side Dish, President's Choice® Blue Menu™	46	¼ pack	36	16	low
Rice & Lentils Espana Side Dish, President's Choice® Blue Menu™	49	¼ pack	36	17	low
Quick cooking brown rice, boiled	80	¾ cup	38	31	high
Uncle Ben's Converted®, white boiled 20–30 min	38	1 cup	36	14	low
Uncle Ben's Converted®, white, long grain boiled 20–30 min	50	1 cup	36	18	low
Wild rice, boiled	57	¾ cup	32	18	med

SNACK FOODS (including nuts and seeds)

Food	GI Value	Nominal Serving Size	Available Carbs	GL Value	GI Level
Apple Cinnamon Soy Chips, NutriSystem®	36	1 oz	10	4	low
Apricot-filled fruit bar, made with whole grain flour ■	50	1.75 oz	34	17	low
Blueberry Dessert Bar, NutriSystem®	36	1.5 oz	21	8	low
Caramel Dessert Bar, NutriSystem®	35	1 oz	21	7	low
Cheese curls, cheese-flavored snack ■	74	1.75 oz	29	22	high
Chocolate, Cadbury's® Milk Chocolate, plain ■	49	1 oz	17	8	low
Chocolate, Dark chocolate, plain ■	41	1 oz	19	8	low
Chocolate, Dove®, milk chocolate ■	45	1.5 oz	29	13	low
Chocolate, Milk chocolate, plain, with fructose instead of sugar ■	20	1 oz	19	4	low
Chocolate, Milk chocolate bar, Nestle® ■	40	2 oz	29	12	low

★ little or no carbohydrate   ■ high in saturated fat   Ⓖ program participant

SNACK FOODS (including nuts and seeds)

Food	GI Value	Nominal Serving Size	Available Carbs	GL Value	GI Level
Chocolate, NutriCrunch Chocolates, NutriSystem®	42	1 oz	15	6	low
Chocolate, white chocolate, plain	44	1.75 oz	29	13	low
Chocolate Chip Granola Bar, NutriSystem®	42	1.4 oz	19	8	low
Chocolate hazelnut spread, Nutella®	30	1 Tbsp.	12	4	low
Chocolate Peanut Butter Bar, NutriSystem®	48	1.5 oz	18	9	low
Chocolate Raspberry Dessert Bar, NutriSystem®	32	1.8 oz	23	7	low
Corn chips, plain, salted	42	1.75 oz	25	11	low
Fudge Graham Lunch Bar, NutriSystem®	33	1.8 oz	23	8	low
Gummi confectionery, made with glucose syrup	94	1.75 oz	36	34	high
Jelly beans	78	1 oz	28	22	high
Licorice, soft	78	2 oz	42	33	high
Life Savers®, peppermint	70	1 oz	30	21	high
M&M's®, peanut ■	33	1 oz	17	6	low
Mars Bar®, regular ■	62	2 oz	40	25	med
Marshmallows, plain, white	62	1 oz	20	12	med
Muesli bar, chewy, with choc chips or fruit	54	1 oz	21	12	low
Muesli bar, crunchy, with dried fruit	61	1 oz	21	13	med
Nuts, Cashews, salted	22	1 oz	9	2	low
Nuts, Peanuts, roasted, salted	14	1.75 oz	6	1	low
Nuts, Pecans, raw	10	1.75 oz	3	1	low
Pop-Tarts®, chocolate	70	1.75 oz	36	25	high
Popcorn, Caramel Pop Corn, NutriSystem®	★	1 oz	8	4	
Popcorn, Microwave Popping Corn, Natural Flavor, President's Choice® Blue Menu™	58	½ bag	26	15	med
Popcorn, plain, popped	72	2 cups	11	8	high
Potato chips, plain, salted ■	54	1.75 oz	18	10	low
Potato crisps, plain, salted ■	54	1.75 oz	18	10	low
Power Bar®, chocolate	56	2 oz	42	24	med
Pretzels, Cheese and Garlic Pretzels, NutriSystem®	34	1 oz	6	2	low
Pretzels, Honey Mustard Pretzels, NutriSystem®	32	1 oz	7	2	low
Pretzels, oven-baked, wheat flour	83	1 oz	20	16	high
Pretzels, Soy Pretzels, NutriSystem®	32	1 oz	7	2	low

★ little or no carbohydrate   ■ high in saturated fat   Ⓖ program participant

SNACK FOODS (including nuts and seeds)

Food	GI Value	Nominal Serving Size	Available Carbs	GL Value	GI Level
Pudding, chocolate, instant, package mix, with whole milk ■	47	½ cup	16	7	low
Pudding, vanilla, instant, package mix with whole milk ■	40	½ cup	16	6	low
Rice Krispies Treat® bar, Kellogg's®	63	1 oz	24	15	med
Roll-Ups®, processed fruit snack	99	1 oz	25	24	high
Sesame seeds	★	2 Tbsp.	0	0	
Skittles® ■	70	1.75 oz	45	32	high
Snickers Bar®, regular ■	41	2 oz	36	15	low
Sour Cream and Onion Soy Chips, NutriSystem®	41	1 oz	10	4	low
Trim Advantage® meal replacement bar, Quixtar	23	1 bar	24	6	low
Twix® bar ■	44	2 oz	39	17	low
White Cheddar Soy Chips, NutriSystem®	38	1 oz	11	4	low

SOUPS

Food	GI Value	Nominal Serving Size	Available Carbs	GL Value	GI Level
Barley Vegetable Low Fat Instant Soup Cup, President's Choice® Blue Menu™	41	1 package	28	11	low
Black bean, canned	64	1 cup	27	17	med
Clear consommé, chicken or vegetable	★	1 cup	0	0	
Green pea, canned	66	1 cup	41	27	med
Lentil, canned	44	1 cup	21	9	low
Minestrone, traditional	39	1 cup	18	7	low
Minestrone & Pasta Low Fat Instant Soup Cup, President's Choice® Blue Menu™	54	1 package	41	22	low

★ little or no carbohydrate　　■ high in saturated fat　　Ⓖ program participant

SOUPS

Food	GI Value	Nominal Serving Size	Available Carbs	GL Value	GI Level
Mushroom Barley Soup, Ready-to-Serve, President's Choice® Blue Menu™	45	1 cup	9	4	low
Pasta E Fagioli Soup, Ready-to-Serve, President's Choice® Blue Menu™	52	1 cup	20	10	low
Pumpkin, creamy	76	1 cup	20	14	high
Soba noodles, instant, served in soup	46	1¼ cups	49	22	low
Split pea, canned	60	1 cup	27	16	med
Spicy Black Bean Low Fat Instant Soup Cup, President's Choice® Blue Menu™	57	1 package	32	18	med
Spicy Thai Instant Noodles with Vegetables Low Fat Instant Soup, Ready-to-Serve, President's Choice® Blue Menu™	56	1 package	31	17	med
Tomato, canned	45	1 cup	17	6	low
Vegetarian Chili Low Fat Instant Cup, President's Choice® Blue Menu™	36	1 package	29	10	low
Vegetarian Chili, Ready-to-Serve, President's Choice® Blue Menu™	39	1 cup	29	11	low
Vegetable Couscous Low Fat Instant Soup Cup, President's Choice® Blue Menu™	57	1 package	33	19	med

★ little or no carbohydrate   ▓ high in saturated fat   Ⓖ program participant

SOY PRODUCTS

Food	GI Value	Nominal Serving Size	Available Carbs	GL Value	GI Level
Apple Cinnamon Soy Chips, NutriSystem®	36	1 oz	10	4	low
Cheese and Garlic Pretzels, NutriSystem®	34	1 oz	6	2	low
Honey Mustard Pretzels, NutriSystem®	32	1 oz	7	2	low
Sour Cream and Onion Soy Chips, NutriSystem®	41	1 oz	10	4	low
Soy Beverage, Original, President's Choice® Blue Menu™	15	8 fl oz	9	1	low
Soy Beverage, Chocolate, President's Choice® Blue Menu™	40	8 fl oz	28	11	low
Soy Beverage, Vanilla, President's Choice® Blue Menu™	28	8 fl oz	16	4	low
Soy milk, full fat, calcium-fortified	36	8 fl oz	18	6	low
Soy milk, reduced-fat, calcium-fortified	44	8 fl oz	17	8	low
Soy Pretzels, NutriSystem®	32	1 oz	7	2	low
Soy smoothie drink, banana, low-fat	30	8 fl oz	22	7	low
Soy yogurt, fruited, 2% fat, with sugar	50	7 oz	26	13	low
White Cheddar Soy Chips, NutriSystem®	38	1 oz	11	4	low

SPREADS & SWEETENERS

Food	GI Value	Nominal Serving Size	Available Carbs	GL Value	GI Level
Ⓖ Agave Nectar, Sweet Cactus Farms	19	1 tsp.	3	1	low
Apricot fruit spread, reduced sugar	55	2 Tbsp.	13	7	low
Avocado	★	2 Tbsp.	0	0	
Chocolate hazelnut spread, Nutella®	30	1 Tbsp.	12	4	low
Diet jelly	★	2 Tbsp.	0	0	
Fructose, pure	19	1 Tbsp.	10	2	low
Golden syrup	63	1 Tbsp.	17	11	med
Honey, 100% pure floral	35	1 Tbsp.	18	6	low
Honey, commercial-blend	64	1 Tbsp.	17	11	med
Honey, various (averaged)	55	1 Tbsp.	18	10	low

★ little or no carbohydrate   ▦ high in saturated fat   Ⓖ program participant

SPREADS & SWEETENERS

Food	GI Value	Nominal Serving Size	Available Carbs	GL Value	GI Level
Hummus, regular	6	2 Tbsp.	5	1	low
Jam, Apricot, 100% fruit	50	1½ Tbsp.	9	4	low
Jam, Blackberry, 100% fruit	46	1½ Tbsp.	9	4	low
Jam, Raspberry, 100% fruit	46	1½ Tbsp.	9	4	low
Jam, Strawberry, 100% fruit	46	1½ Tbsp.	9	4	low
Maple flavored syrup	68	1 Tbsp.	22	15	med
Maple syrup, pure, Canadian	54	1 Tbsp.	18	10	low
Marmalade, orange	55	1½ Tbsp.	20	9	low
Nutella®, hazlenut spread	33	1 Tbsp.	12	4	low
Sugar, granulated, white	60	1 Tbsp.	10	7	med
Vinegar	★	2 Tbsp.	0	0	

VEGETABLES

Food	GI Value	Nominal Serving Size	Available Carbs	GL Value	GI Level
Alfalfa sprouts, raw	★	½ cup	0	0	
Artichokes, globe, fresh or canned	★	½ cup	0	0	
Arugula, raw	★	1 cup	0	0	
Asparagus	★	½ cup	0	0	
Bean sprouts	★	½ cup	0	0	
Beets, red, canned	64	½ cup	7	5	med
Bok choy	★	½ cup	0	0	
Broad beans (fava)	79	½ cup	11	9	high
Broccoli	★	½ cup	0	0	
Brussels sprouts	★	½ cup	0	0	
Cabbage	★	½ cup	0	0	
Carrots, cooked	41	½ cup	5	2	low
Cauliflower	★	½ cup	0	0	
Celery	★	½ cup	0	0	
Chili peppers, fresh or dried	★	1 Tsp.	0	0	
Chives, fresh	★	2 Tbsp.	0	0	
Corn, sweet, on the cob	48	1 med ear	16	8	low
Corn, sweet, whole kernel, canned	46	⅓ cup	14	7	low

★ little or no carbohydrate   ▦ high in saturated fat   Ⓖ program participant

VEGETABLES

Food	GI Value	Nominal Serving Size	Available Carbs	GL Value	GI Level
Cucumber	★	½ cup	0	0	
Eggplant	★	½ cup	0	0	
Endive	★	1 cup	0	0	
Fennel	★	½ cup	0	0	
Garlic	★	1 clove	0	0	
Ginger	★	1 Tsp.	0	0	
Green beans	★	½ cup	0	0	
Herbs, fresh or dried	★	2 Tbsp.	0	0	
Leeks	★	½ cup	0	0	
Lettuce	★	1 cup	0	0	
Mushrooms	★	½ cup	0	0	
Okra	★	½ cup	0	0	
Onions	★	½ cup	0	0	
Parsnips	97	½ cup	12	12	high
Peas, green	48	½ cup	7	3	low
Peppers	★	½ cup	0	0	
Potato, average, boiled	72	1 med (5 oz)	18	16	high
Potato, average, microwaved	79	1 med (5 oz)	18	14	high
Potato, french fries, frozen, reheated ■	75	5 oz	29	22	high
Potato, instant, mashed	88	¾ cup	20	18	high
Potato, new, canned	65	6 sm (5 oz)	18	12	med
Potato, russet, baked without fat	77	1 med (5 oz)	30	23	high
Radishes	★	½ cup	0	0	
Scallions	★	2 Tbsp.	0	0	
Shallots	★	2 Tbsp.	0	0	
Snow pea sprouts	★	½ cup	0	0	
Spinach	★	1 cup	0	0	
Squash, yellow	★	½ cup	0	0	
Sweet potato	46	1 med (5 oz)	25	11	low
Swiss chard	★	1 cup	0	0	
Taro	54	¼ cup	8	4	low
Tomato	★	½ cup	0	0	
Turnip	★	½ cup	0	0	
Watercress	★	1 cup	0	0	
Yam	37	1 med (5 oz)	36	13	low
Zucchini	★	½ cup	0	0	

★ little or no carbohydrate   ■ high in saturated fat   Ⓖ program participant

Glossary
An A to Z of Key Terms Used Throughout This Book

A1c (also called **HbA1c**, **hemoglobin A1c**, or **glycosylated or glycolated hemoglobin**) a blood test that measures your average blood glucose level over the previous 2–3 months. It indicates the percentage of hemoglobin (the part of the red blood cell that carries oxygen to the cells and sometimes joins with glucose in the bloodstream) that is "glycated." *Glycated* means it has a glucose molecule riding on its back. This is proportional to the amount of glucose in the blood. The higher the level of HbA1c, the greater the risk of developing diabetic complications. If you have diabetes, it should be measured 2–4 times a year, depending on your type, and you should aim to keep it under 7 percent.

Alternative sweeteners include nutritive sweeteners (which add calories to the diet) and nonnutritive sweeteners, which are calorie free. *Nutritive sweeteners,* including sugars, sugar-alcohols, and oligosaccharides (medium-sized chains of glucose), are simply different types of carbohydrate with varying levels of sweetness. The sugar alcohols sorbitol, mannitol, and maltitol are generally not as sweet as table sugar, provide fewer calories, and have less of an impact on blood glucose levels.

Non-nutritive sweeteners (such as Equal, Splenda, Stevia, NutraSweet, or saccharin, for example) are all much sweeter than table sugar and have essentially no effect on your blood glucose levels because most are used in such small quantities and are not absorbed into or metabolized by the body. Because they are used in only minute amounts, the number of calories they provide is insignificant. Nonnutritive sweeteners made of protein molecules often break down when heated for long periods and lose their sweetness.

Area under the curve refers, in the context of the GI testing of food, to the blood glucose response to a test food when it is plotted on a graph and compared with the response to the reference food.

Atherosclerosis, or hardening of the arteries, is a slow, progressive disease that produces problems such as angina, heart attack, or stroke. Most heart disease is caused by atherosclerosis—clogging on the inside wall of the arteries through the slow buildup of fatty deposits (called plaque) that narrow the arteries and reduce the blood flow. If the plaque ruptures, clots form, causing a more acute, total blockage. If the blood vessel is providing blood to the heart, the result is a heart attack. Atherosclerosis can affect the arteries to the heart and in the brain, kidneys, and the arms and legs.

Autoimmune disease is a disorder in which the body's immune system mistakenly attacks and destroys body tissue or organs that it believes to be foreign; type 1 diabetes (see below) is an autoimmune condition.

Beta cells produce the hormone insulin. They are found grouped together in the Islets of Langerhans in the pancreas.

Blood glucose (blood sugar or **glucose**) is the most common kind of sugar found in the blood and is the main source of energy for most of the body's organs and tissues and the only source of fuel for the brain. When the body's digestive organs process carbohydrates, the food ends up as glucose, which passes through the walls of the intestine into the bloodstream to the liver and eventually into general circulation. From here the glucose enters individual cells or tissues throughout the body to be used for fuel and provide energy.

Blood glucose level (BGL) is the amount of glucose in the bloodstream. If you haven't eaten in the past few hours (and you don't have diabetes), your blood glucose level will normally fall within the range of 70–110 mg/dL (3.9–6 mmol/L). If you eat, this will rise, but rarely above 180 mg/dL (10 mmol/L). The extent of the increase will vary depending on your glucose tolerance (your own physiological response) and the type of food you have just eaten.

Blood pressure is the pressure of the blood on the inside walls of your blood vessels caused by the beating of the heart. It is expressed as a ratio such as "120/80." The first number is the *systolic* pressure, or the pressure when the heart pushes the blood out into the arteries. The second number is the *diastolic* pressure, or the pressure when the heart rests between beats. High blood pressure (or hypertension), above 140/90, is the most common cardiovascular disease risk factor. High blood pressure is more common in people with diabetes and increases the risk of stroke, heart attack, and diseases of the kidney and eye. Your blood pressure should be measured when you visit your doctor for checkups or at least twice a year, with a goal of 130/80 mm Hg or lower.

Blood sugar. See **blood glucose**.

BMI (Body Mass Index) is a measure that evaluates body relative to height to find out if an individual is underweight, in the healthy weight range, overweight, or obese. It has limitations: it can overestimate body fat in athletes and others who have a muscular build, such as body builders, and in pregnant women, and it can underestimate body fat in older people or people with a disability who have lost muscle mass. It's not appropriate for children and young people under eighteen. For an easy online calculator, go to www.nhlbisupport.com/bmi/

BMI categories:

Less than 18.5	Underweight
18.5–24.9	Healthy weight range
25–29.9	Overweight
Over 30	Obese

For Maori and Pacific Island people: BMI is 20–26 for the healthy weight range, 27–31 for overweight, and over 32 for obese.

Calorie (or kilocalorie, to be technically correct) is the unit that measures the energy you get from the food you eat (your energy intake). Carbohydrate, protein, fat, and alcohol all provide calories in your diet. Carbs and protein provide 4 calories per gram, fat 9 calories per gram, and alcohol 7. A kilocalorie is the amount of energy (or heat) needed to increase the temperature of one kilogram of water by 1°C. The equivalent metric unit is the *kilojoule* (kJ). You can convert calories to kilojoules by multiplying by 4.2; you can convert kilojoules to calories by dividing by 4.2.

Carbohydrate is one of the three main macronutrients in food; protein and fat are the other two. Carbohydrate is the starchy part of foods like rice, bread, legumes, potatoes, and pasta, and the sugars in foods like fruit, milk, and honey, and certain types of fiber. Some foods contain a large amount of carbohydrate (cereals, potatoes, sweet potatoes, yams, taro, and legumes), while other foods, such as carrots, broccoli, and salad vegetables, are very dilute sources. *See also* **fiber**, **starch**, and **sugars**.

Carbohydrate counting is a method of meal planning for people with diabetes based on counting the grams of carbohydrate in food.

Carbohydrate exchange is an amount of food typically containing an average of 15 (12–17) grams of carbohydrate. It is one of several approaches to meal planning for people with diabetes. Lists set out the serving sizes of different carb foods and assign a certain number of exchanges to each meal over the course of the day. The system is intended to promote consistency in the amount of carbohydrate eaten from day to day. It was developed long before research on the glycemic index was published, and thus the emphasis is purely on carbohydrate quantity rather than carbohydrate quality.

Cardiovascular disease, or CVD, refers to the diseases that involve the heart and/or blood vessels (arteries and veins), particularly those related to atherosclerosis in the heart, brain, and lower limbs.

Cardiovascular system is the heart and blood vessels. It is the means by which blood is pumped from the heart and circulated through the body. As the blood circulates, it carries nourishment and oxygen to all the body's tissues. It also removes waste products.

Celiac disease is a condition in which the lining of the small intestine is damaged due to an immune reaction from the body to gluten, a small protein. Gluten is found in certain grain foods, such as wheat, rye, triticale (a hybrid of wheat and rye), and barley, and in much smaller amounts in oats (as a contaminant). The only treatment for celiac disease at present is a gluten-free diet.

Central obesity, or your waist measurement, is often a better predictor of your health risks than BMI. Abdominal fat increases your risk of heart disease, high blood pressure, and diabetes. The cutoff waist measurements are:

For people of Caucasian (European) origin:
Men   37 inches (94 cm)
Women   31.5 inches (80 cm)
For people from South Asia, China and Japan:
Men   90 cm/35.5 inches
Women   80 cm/31.1 inches
Until more specific data are available:
Ethnic South and Central Americans should use South Asian data.
Sub-Saharan Africans should use European data.
Eastern Mediterranean and Middle East (Arab) populations should use European data.

Cholesterol is a soft waxy substance found in the blood and in all the body's cells. It is an important part of a healthy body because it is part of the walls around all the body's cells and is a major component of many of the hormones the body produces. Most of the cholesterol the body needs is manufactured by the liver. It is also found in some animal foods (eggs, milk, cheese, liver, meat, and poultry). High levels of cholesterol in the blood can lead to blocked arteries, heart attack, and stroke. Cholesterol and other fats can't dissolve in the blood. They have to be transported to and from the cells by special carriers called *lipoproteins*. The most common ones are low-density lipoprotein (LDL) cholesterol and high-density lipoprotein (HDL) cholesterol.

HDL cholesterol is known as "good" cholesterol because higher levels of HDL seem to protect against heart attack and stroke. HDL tends to sweep excess cholesterol from the blood back to the liver, where it is eliminated from the body.

LDL cholesterol is the main form of cholesterol in the blood and does most of the damage to blood vessels; it's a red flag for cardiovascular disease. If there is too much LDL cholesterol in the blood, it can slowly build up in the walls of the blood vessels that feed the heart, brain and other important organs, causing a heart attack or stroke.

Recommended ranges for people with diabetes:
Total cholesterol   <200 mg/dL (<5.1 mmol/L)
Triglycerides   <150 mg/dL (<1.7 mmol/L)
HDL cholesterol
    men: >40 mg/dL (>1.0 mmol/L)

women: >50 mg/dL (>1.3 mmol/L)
LDL cholesterol <100 mg/dL (<2.5 mmol/L)
Total cholesterol/HDL ratio men: <5.0; women: <4.0

Complications are the harmful effects of diabetes, including damage to the blood vessels, heart, nervous system, eyes, feet, kidneys, teeth, and gums. Studies show that keeping blood glucose, blood pressure, and cholesterol levels within the recommended ranges can help to prevent or delay these problems.

Diabetes

Type 1 diabetes is characterized by high blood glucose levels due to the body's complete inability to produce insulin. It occurs when the body's immune system attacks the insulin-producing beta cells in the pancreas and destroys them. The pancreas then produces very little or no insulin. Type 1 diabetes occurs most often in young people but can develop in adults.

Type 2 diabetes is characterized by high blood glucose levels caused by an insufficiency of insulin and the body's inability to use insulin efficiently. It is thought to occur when the body becomes **insulin resistant**. The pancreas compensates initially by producing more insulin, then eventually becomes exhausted and doesn't produce enough insulin. Type 2 diabetes occurs most often in middle-aged and older people but is being seen increasingly in younger people—even adolescents. See also **gestational diabetes**.

Energy The foods we eat provide energy (fuel for the body), which is measured in kilojoules or calories. Just how much energy a food provides depends on the amount of carbohydrate, protein, and fat it contains. The technical term for this used to be "calorie," but "kilojoule" tends now to be accepted internationally. The terms *calorie* and *kilojoule* allow us to talk about how much energy a food contains and how much energy is burned up during exercise.

Energy density The number of calories in a food, per gram or per serving size.

Fasting blood glucose is a blood test in which a sample of your blood is drawn after an overnight fast (8–12 hours) to measure the amount of glucose in your blood. The test is used to diagnose diabetes and prediabetes and to monitor people who already have type 2 diabetes.

Fat is one of the three main nutrients in food and provides 9 calories, or 37 kilojoules, per gram. Today's health message is to focus on the good fats (mono- and polyunsaturated fats) and avoid the bad fats (trans fats and saturated fats). You don't actually need to eat any saturated fat, since the body can make all it requires, but it is fairly difficult not to eat some, since all fats are actually mixtures of saturated and unsaturated fats.

Saturated fats are solid or semisolid at room temperature. These are the fats on meat, and in chicken skin, butter, cheese, palm oil, and coconut oil. Saturated fats raise blood cholesterol levels by increasing the amount of cholesterol produced by the liver, causing it to build up in the bloodstream and become part of the plaque that forms on the walls of the blood vessels.

Monounsaturated fat is a type of unsaturated fat that comes from plant foods. It's considered to be the "healthiest" of all fats; in fact, studies show that it can boost levels of good HDL cholesterol and that a diet rich in monounsaturated fats may reduce the risk of heart disease. Sources include olive oil, canola oil, peanuts, and olives.

Polyunsaturated fat is a type of unsaturated fat that comes from fish and plant foods. It's considered to be healthier than saturated fat, but it lowers levels of both bad LDL cholesterol *and* good HDL cholesterol. Sources include safflower, sunflower, soybean, corn, and cottonseed oils, as well as salmon, tuna, and other fish.

Transfatty acids or *trans fats* occur naturally in small amounts in the fat of dairy products and meat. They are also formed by hydrogenation—a chemical process that changes a liquid oil into a solid fat. Foods high in trans fats include fried fast foods, some margarines, crackers, cookies, and snack foods. The United States now requires that food manufacturers list the amount of trans fat in the Nutrition Facts panel on the label. Trans fats can raise cholesterol levels and are linked with an increased risk of **cardiovascular disease**.

Fatty liver disease is the buildup of excessive amounts of triglycerides and other fats inside liver cells; also known as *steatohepatitis* or *NASH* (Nonalcoholic Steatohepatitis).

Fiber Dietary fibers are mainly carbohydrate molecules made up of many different sorts of *monosaccharides*. They are different from starches and sugars in that they are not broken down by human digestive enzymes, and they reach the large intestine largely unchanged. Once there, bacteria begin to ferment and break down the fibers. Dietary fiber comes mainly from the outer bran layers of grains (corn, oats, wheat, and rice, and in foods containing these grains), fruits and vegetables, and nuts and legumes (dried beans, peas, and lentils). There are three main types of fiber—soluble, insoluble, and resistant starch.

Soluble fibers can be dissolved in water—the gel, gum, and often jellylike components of apples, oats, and legumes. Some soluble fibers are very viscous when in solution. By slowing down the time it takes for food to pass through the stomach and small intestine, soluble fiber can lower the glycemic response to a food. Good sources include oatmeal, oat bran, nuts and seeds, legumes (beans, peas, and lentils), apples, pears, strawberries, and blueberries.

Insoluble fibers such as cellulose, are insoluble, meaning they are not soluble in water and do not directly affect the speed of digestion. They are dry and branlike and are commonly called *roughage*. All cereal grains and products that retain the outer coat of the grain they are made from are sources of insoluble fiber, e.g., whole-wheat bread and All-Bran, but not all foods containing insoluble fiber are low GI. Insoluble fibers will only lower the GI of a food when they exist in their original, intact form; for example, in whole grains of wheat. Here they act as a physical barrier, delaying access of digestive enzymes and water to the starch within the cereal grain. Good sources include whole grains, whole-wheat breads, barley, couscous, brown rice, bulghur, wheat bran, seeds, and most vegetables.

Resistant starch. See page 328.

Fructose. See **sugars**.

Fuel hierarchy The body runs on fuel the way a car runs on gasoline. The fuels the body burns are derived from a mixture of the protein, fat, carbohydrate, and alcohol you consume. The fuel hierarchy describes the priority for burning the fuels in food. Alcohol is burned first, because the body has no place to store unused alcohol and it is potentially toxic to many of the body's organs and tissues. Protein comes second, followed by carbohydrate, while fat is last in line. In practice, the fuel mix is usually a combination of carbohydrate and fat in varying proportions—after meals the mix is mainly carbohydrate; before meals it is mainly fat.

Gestational diabetes can develop during pregnancy but usually goes away after the baby is born. Hormones released by the placenta during pregnancy reduce the effectiveness of the mother's insulin.

It is usually managed successfully with healthy eating and regular physical activity. Some women may require insulin as well.

Glucose is a simple form of sugar (a *monosaccharide*) that is created when the body's digestive processes break down the carbohydrate foods you eat such as bread, cereals, and fruit. It is this glucose that is absorbed from the intestine and becomes the fuel that circulates in the bloodstream.

Glucose tolerance test (GTT) a test used in the diagnosis of diabetes and prediabetes. Glucose in the blood is measured at regular intervals for a couple of hours before and after a person has drunk either 50 or 75 g of pure glucose, after an overnight fast.

Glycemia is the concentration of glucose in the blood. Hence the adjective **glycemic**.

Glycemic index (GI) Different carbohydrate foods can behave quite differently in the body. Some break down quickly during digestion and release glucose rapidly into the bloodstream; others break down gradually and slowly trickle glucose into the blood stream. The glycemic index, or GI, is a numerical ranking on a scale of 0 to 100 that describes this difference. It is a measure of carbohydrate quality. After testing hundreds of carbohydrate foods around the world, scientists have found that foods with a low GI will have less effect on your blood glucose than foods with a high GI. High-GI foods tend to cause spikes in your glucose levels, whereas low-GI foods tend to cause gentle increases. All foods are compared with a reference food and tested using an internationally standardized method.

Glycemic Index Symbol Program is a program that encourages manufacturers to have their carbohydrate foods GI tested at an accredited laboratory and to list the results on the labels of their foods. Foods that are part of the GISP must meet strict nutrition criteria to ensure that they are healthy foods. They are easily identified by the program's distinct logo. More details can be found at the program's Web site, www.gisymbol.com.

Glycemic load (GL) How much your blood glucose actually increases and how long it remains high when you eat a meal containing carbohydrate depends on both the quality of the carbohydrate (its GI) and the quantity of carbohydrate in the meal. Researchers at Harvard University came up with a term to describe this: glycemic load. It is calculated by multiplying the GI of a food by the available carbohydrate content (carbohydrate minus fiber) in the serving (expressed in grams), divided by 100 (GL = GI ÷ 100 × available carbs per serving).

Glycemic response or **glycemic impact** describes the change or pattern of change in blood glucose after you have consumed a food or a meal. Glucose responses can be fast or slow, short or prolonged. It is primarily determined by the food's carbohydrate content. Other factors include how much food you eat, how much the food is processed, and even how the food is prepared (for example, pasta that is cooked al dente has a slower glycemic response than pasta that is overcooked).

Glycosylated hemoglobin. See **A1c**.

Gram is a unit of weight in the metric system. one ounce equals 28 grams (often rounded up to 30). One typical slice of bread is 30 grams.

Glycogen is the name given to the glucose stores in the body. It can be readily broken down into glucose to maintain normal blood glucose levels. Approximately 60 percent of the body's glycogen is found in the muscles and 40 percent in the liver. The total stores of glycogen in the body are relatively small, however, and will be exhausted in about twenty-four hours during fasting or starvation.

HbA1c. See **A1c**.

HDL cholesterol. See **cholesterol**.

High blood glucose. See **hyperglycemia**.

Hormones are "chemical messengers" made in one part of the body and released into the bloodstream to trigger or regulate particular functions of another part of the body. For example, insulin is a hormone made in the pancreas that lets glucose into cells throughout the body so that they can produce energy.

Hyperglycemia is a condition that occurs when there are excessively high levels of glucose in the blood. The symptoms usually occur when blood glucose levels go above 270 mg/dL (15 mmol/L), and include extreme thirst, frequent urination and large volumes of urine, weakness, and weight loss. If left untreated it can lead to the production of *ketones*, deep breathing, abdominal pain, drowsiness, and eventually unconsciousness, coma, and death.

Hyperinsulinemia is a condition when the level of insulin in the blood is higher than normal. It is caused by overproduction of insulin by the body and is related to **insulin resistance**.

Hypertension. See **blood pressure**.

Hypoglycemia (also called an insulin reaction) occurs when a person's blood glucose falls below normal levels—usually less than 70 mg/dL (3.9 mmol/L). It is treated by consuming a carb-rich food, such as a glucose tablet or juice. It may also be treated with an injection of *glucagon* if the person is unconscious or unable to swallow. See also **reactive hypoglycemia**.

Immune system is the body's defense system, which protects itself from viruses, bacteria, and any "foreign" substances.

Impaired fasting glucose is a condition in which the fasting blood glucose level is elevated (100–125 mg/dL; 5.6–6.9 mmol/L) after an overnight fast but is not high enough to be classified as diabetes. It is sometimes called **prediabetes**.

Impaired glucose tolerance is a condition in which the blood sugar level is elevated (140–199 mg/dL; 7.8–11 mmol/L or) after a two–hour oral glucose tolerance test but is not high enough to be classified as diabetes. It is now called **prediabetes**. People with impaired glucose tolerance are at increased risk of developing diabetes, heart disease, and stroke.

Insulin is a hormone produced by the pancreas that helps glucose pass into the cells, where it is used to create energy for the body. The pancreas should automatically produce the right amount of insulin to move glucose into the cells. When the body cannot make enough insulin, it has to be taken by injection or through use of an insulin pump. It can't be taken by mouth, because it will be broken down by the body's digestive juices. Insulin is not only involved in regulating blood glucose levels, but it also plays a key part in determining whether we burn fat or carbohydrate to meet our energy needs— it switches muscle cells from fat burning to carb burning. For this reason, lowering insulin levels is one of the secrets to lifelong health.

Insulinemia simply means the presence of insulin in the blood; hyperinsulinemia is excessive amounts of insulin in the blood.

Insulin resistance means that your muscle and liver cells are not good at taking up glucose unless there's a lot of insulin around. Chances are you'll have very high insulin levels even long after a meal, as the body tries to metabolize the carbohydrate in the meal. When insulin levels in the body are chronically raised, the cells that usually respond to insulin become resistant to its signals. The body then responds by secreting more and more insulin, a never-ending vicious cycle that spells trouble on many fronts. Insulin resistance is at the root of prediabetes and type 2 diabetes, many forms of heart disease, and polycystic ovarian syndrome (PCOS).

Insulin resistance syndrome. See **metabolic syndrome**.

Insulin sensitivity If you are insulin sensitive, your muscle and liver cells take up glucose rapidly without the need for a lot of insulin. Exercise keeps you insulin sensitive; so does a moderately high carbohydrate intake.

Ketones are the breakdown products of fat, which some of the body's cells can use for fuel. They occur in higher concentrations when the body is unable to use glucose as a fuel due to insufficient insulin. Ketones are strong acids, and when they are produced in large quantities they can upset the body's delicate acid-base balance. They are normally released into the urine, but if levels are very high or if the person is dehydrated, they may begin to build up in the blood. High blood levels of ketones may cause fruity-smelling breath, loss of appetite, nausea or vomiting, fast, deep breathing (to blow off the acid in the form of carbon dioxide), and excessive urination (to eliminate the extra acid). In severe cases, it may lead to coma and death. In a pregnant woman, even a moderate amount of ketones in the blood may harm the baby and impair brain development. The excessive formation of ketones in the blood is called *ketosis*. Large amounts of ketones in the urine may signal *diabetic ketoacidosis*, a dangerous condition that is caused by very high blood glucose levels.

Ketosis is the metabolic state in which the body is burning fat for fuel. Normally, carbohydrates are the main source of fuel for your brain and nervous system, kidneys, and many other organs.

Kilojoule (kJ) is the metric system for measuring the amount of energy produced when food is completely metabolized in the body. The *calorie* is the imperial (official British) measure of energy, and can be calculated from the number of kilojoules by dividing by 4.2.

LDL cholesterol. See **cholesterol**.

Lipid profile is a blood test that measures total cholesterol, triglycerides, and HDL cholesterol. LDL cholesterol is then usually calculated from the results, though it can sometimes be measured separately. Your lipid profile is one measure of your risk of cardiovascular disease.

Lipids is a term for fat in the body. The most common lipids are cholesterol and triglycerides (sometimes called triacylglycerols).

Macronutrients are the three main components in foods: **carbohydrate**, **protein**, and **fat**.

Metabolic syndrome is a cluster of serious heart disease risk factors. A person with metabolic syndrome will have central or abdominal obesity plus two of the following risk factors: high triglycerides, low HDL cholesterol, raised blood pressure, raised blood glucose. Tests on patients with the metabolic syndrome show that insulin resistance is very common.

Metabolism is the term used to describe how the cells of the body chemically change the food you consume and make the protein, fats, and carbohydrates into forms of energy or use them for growth and repair.

mg/dL stands for milligrams per deciliter—a unit of measure that shows the concentration of a substance in a specific amount of fluid. In the United States, blood glucose test results are reported as mg/dL. Medical journals and other countries, including Canada, use millimoles per liter (mmol/L). To convert blood glucose levels to mg/dL from mmol/L, multiply mmol/L by 18. Example: 10 mmol/L $\times$ 18 = 180 mg/dL.

mmol/L stands for millimoles per liter—a unit of measure that shows the concentration of a substance in a specific amount of fluid. In most of the world, including Canada, blood glucose test results are reported as mmol/L. In the United States, milligrams per deciliter (mg/dL) is used. To convert blood glucose results to mmol/L from mg/dL, divide mg/dL $\times$ 18. Example: 180 mg/dL $\div$ 18 = 10 mmol/L.

Monounsaturated fat. See **fats**.

Nurses' Health Study Established in 1976 by Dr. Frank Speizer at Harvard's Channing Laboratory, one of the largest ongoing studies of the risk factors in women for developing major chronic diseases. The study follows registered nurses, because due to their medical background, they can easily and accurately answer specific, health-related questions. Every two years, more than 100,000 nurses provide personal information about diseases and health, including diet and nutrition, smoking, hormones, and general quality of life. The study is now conducted under the aegis of the Harvard School of Public Health.

Obesity is defined as when a person's BMI is > 30 kg/m2. The risk of developing prediabetes, type 2 diabetes, heart disease, stroke, and arthritis is very high when a person is obese.

Overweight is defined as when a person's BMI is between 25 and 29.9 kg/m2. The healthy weight range is 18.5—24.9 kg/m2. The risk of developing prediabetes, type 2 diabetes, heart disease, and stroke starts to increase when a person is overweight.

Pancreas is a vital organ near the stomach that secretes the digestive juices that help break down food during digestion and produces the hormones insulin and glucagon.

PCOS (polycystic ovarian syndrome) can have a number of different causes. Elements of PCOS are thought to affect one in four women in developed countries. At the root of PCOS is insulin resistance. The signs of PCOS range from subtle symptoms such as faint facial hair to a "full house" syndrome—lack of periods, infertility, heavy body-hair growth, acne or skin pigmentation, obstinate body fat, diabetes, and cardiovascular disease.

Postprandial glucose The increase in blood glucose that occurs immediately after a meal that contains appreciable (> 10 grams per serving) amounts of carbohydrate.

Prediabetes is a condition in which blood glucose levels are higher than normal but not high enough for a diagnosis of diabetes. People with prediabetes may have impaired fasting glucose or impaired glucose tolerance. Some people have both. Studies show that most people with prediabetes will develop type 2 diabetes within ten years if they don't make lifestyle changes such as losing weight, eating a healthy diet, and exercising more. They are also at increased risk of having a heart attack or stroke.

Protein is one of the three main macronutrients from food along with fat and carbohydrate. The body uses protein to build and repair body tissue—muscles, bones, skin, hair, and virtually every other body part are made of protein. The best sources are meat, egg, fish, seafood, poultry, and dairy foods. Other sources are plant proteins—legumes (beans, chickpeas, and lentils), tofu, cereal grains (especially whole grains), and nuts and seeds. Because our bodies can't stockpile amino acids (the building blocks of protein) from one day to the next as it does fat or carbs, we need a daily supply. Women on average need about 45 grams of protein a day (more if they are pregnant or breast-feeding), and men about 55 grams. Active people may need more, as do growing children and teenagers.

Polyunsaturated fat. See **fats**.

Reactive hypoglycemia is the most common form of hypoglycemia, when your blood glucose level rises too quickly after you have eaten, causing the release of too much insulin. This then draws too much glucose out of the blood, your blood glucose levels fall below normal, and you suffer a variety of unpleasant symptoms, including sweating, tremor, anxiety, palpitations, weakness, restlessness, irritability, poor concentration, lethargy, and drowsiness.

Resistant starch is the starch that completely resists digestion in the small intestine. It cannot contribute to the glycemic effect, because it is not absorbed but passes through to the large intestine, where it acts just like dietary fiber to improve bowel health. Sources of resistant starch are foods such as unprocessed cereals and whole grains, firm (unripe) bananas, legumes, potatoes, and especially starchy foods that have been cooked and then cooled (such as cold potatoes or rice, sushi, or pasta salads). Resistant starch is also added to some refined cereal products, including breads and breakfast cereals, to increase their fiber content.

Retinopathy is damage to the retina of the eye caused by high blood glucose and blood pressure. Once a major cause of blindness in people with diabetes, modern laser therapy can now successfully treat many people with this condition.

Risk factor is anything that increases your chances of developing a disease.

Satiety is the feeling of fullness and satisfaction we experience after eating. Carbohydrate-rich foods and protein provide the best satiety.

Saturated fats. See **fats**.

Starches are long chains of sugar molecules. They are called *polysaccharides* (poly meaning many). They are not sweet-tasting. There are two sorts—amylose and amylopectin.

Amylose is a straight-chain molecule, like a string of beads. These tend to line up in rows and form tight, compact clumps that are harder to gelatinize and therefore digest.

Amylopectin is a string of glucose molecules with lots of branching points, such as you see in some types of seaweed. Amylopectin molecules are larger and more open and the starch is easier to gelatinize and digest. See also **resistant starch**.

Starch gelatinization happens when starch granules have swollen and burst during cooking—the starch is said to be fully gelatinized. The starch in raw food is stored in hard, compact granules that make it difficult to digest. Most starchy foods need to be cooked for this reason. During cooking, water and heat expand the starch granules to different degrees; some granules actually burst and free the individual starch molecules. The swollen granules and free starch molecules are very easy to digest, because the starch-digesting enzymes in the small intestine have a greater surface area to attack. A food containing starch that is fully gelatinized will therefore have a very high GI value.

Sugars are a type of carbohydrate. The simplest is a single-sugar molecule called a *monosaccharide* (mono meaning one, saccharide meaning sweet). Glucose is a monosaccharide that occurs in food (as glucose itself and as the building block of starch). If two monosaccharides are joined together, the result is a *disaccharide* (di meaning two). *Sucrose*, or common table sugar, is a disaccharide, as is *lactose*, the sugar in milk. As the number of monosaccharides in the chain increases, the carbohydrate becomes less sweet. Maltodextrins are *oligosaccharides* (oligo meaning a few) that are 5 or 6 glucose residues long and commonly used as a food ingredient. They taste only faintly sweet.

Syndrome X. See **metabolic syndrome**.

Trans fats. See **fats**.

Triglycerides, also known as **triacylglycerols** or **blood fats**, are another type of fat linked to increased risk of heart disease. Having too much triglyceride often goes hand in hand with having too little HDL cholesterol. Having high levels of triglycerides can be inherited, but it's most often associated with being overweight or obese. People with diabetes should aim to keep their triglyceride levels under 150 mg/dL (1.7 mmol/L), as they are at greater risk of cardiovascular disease.

Type 1 diabetes. See **diabetes**.

Type 2 diabetes. See **diabetes**.

Unsaturated fat. See **fats**.

Vasodilation is the normal increase in the diameter of blood vessels that occurs after a meal.

Further Reading:
Sources and References

Agus, M. S. D., J. F. Swain, C. L. Larson, E. A. Eckert, and D. S. Ludwig. 2000. "Dietary composition and physiologic adaptations to energy restriction." *American Journal of Clinical Nutrition* 71:901–07.

Bahadori, B., B. Yazdani-Biuki, P. Krippl, H. Brath, E. Uitz, and T. C. Wascher. 2005. "Low-fat, high-carbohydrate (low-glycaemic index) diet induces weight loss and preserves lean body mass in obese healthy subjects: results of a 24-week study." *Diabetes, Obesity and Metabolism* 7(3):290–93.

American Diabetes Association. 2001. "Nutrition recommendations and principles for people with diabetes mellitus." *Diabetes Care* 24(S1).

Brand-Miller, J. C. 2003. "Glycemic load and chronic disease." *Nutrition Review* 61 (May): S49–55.

Brand-Miller, J. C., and S. Colagiuri. 1999. "Evolutionary aspects of diet and insulin resistance." *World Review of Nutrition and Dietetics* 84:74–105.

Brand-Miller, J. C., S. H. A. Holt, D. B. Pawlak, and J. McMillan. 2002. "Glycemic index and obesity." *American Journal of Clinical Nutrition* 76:281S–285S.

Bruce, W. R., T. M. S. Wolever, and A. Giacca. 2000. "Mechanisms linking diet and colorectal cancer: the possible role of insulin resistance." *Nutrition and Cancer* 37:19–26.

Brynes, A. E., J. L. Lee, R. E. Brighton, A. R. Leeds, A. Dornhorst, and G. S. Frost. 2003. "A low glycemic diet significantly improves the 24-h blood glucose profile in people with type 2 diabetes, as assessed using the continuous glucose MiniMed monitor." *Diabetes Care* 26(2) (Feb.): 548–49.

Buyken, A. E., M. Toeller, G. Heitkamp, B. Karamanos, R. Rottiers, M. Muggeo, J. H. Fuller, and the EURODIAB IDDM Complications Study Group. 2001. "Glycemic index in the diet of European outpatients with type 1 diabetes: relations to glycated hemoglobin and serum lipids." *American Journal of Clinical Nutrition* 73:574–81.

Diabetes and Nutrition Study Group (DNSG) of the European Association for the Study of Diabetes (EASD). 2000. "Recommendations for the nutritional management of patients with diabetes mellitus." *European Journal of Clinical Nutrition* 54:353–55.

Dietitians Association of Australia review paper. 1997. "Glycaemic index in diabetes management." *Australian Journal of Nutrition and Dietetics* 54(2):57–63.

Dumesnil, J. G., J. Turgeon, A. Tremblay, et al. 2001. "Effect of a low-glycaemic index-low-fat-high protein diet on the atherogenic metabolic risk profile of abdominally obese men." *British Journal of Nutrition* 86:557–68.

Food and Agriculture Organisation/World Health Organisation. 1998. "Carbohydrates in Human Nutrition, Report of a Joint FAO/WHO Expert Consultation." Rome, 14–18 April 1997. FAO Food and Nutrition Paper 66.

Ford, E. S., and S. Liu. 2001. "Glycemic index and serum high-density-lipoprotein cholesterol concentration among US adults." *Archives of Internal Medicine* 161:572–76.

Foster-Powell, K., S. H. Holt, and J. C. Brand-Milller. 2002. "International table of glycemic index and glycemic load values: 2002." *American Journal of Clinical Nutrition* 76 (1) (July): 5–56.

Franceschi, S., L. Dal Maso, L. Augustin, E. Negri, M. Parpinel, P. Boyle, D. J. A. Jenkins, and C. La Vecchia. 2001. "Dietary glycemic load and colorectal cancer risk." *Annals of Oncology* 12:1–6.

Frost, G., A. Leeds, D. Dore, S. Madeiros, S. Brading, and A. Dornhorst. 1999. "Glycaemic index as a determinant of serum HDL-cholesterol concentration." *Lancet* 353:1045–48.

Frost, G., and A. Dornhorst. 2000. "The relevance of the glycaemic index to our understanding of dietary carbohydrates." *Diabetic Medicine* 17:336–45.

Frost, G., B. Keogh, D. Smith, K. Akinsanya, and A. R. Leeds. 1996. "The effect of low glycemic carbohydrate on insulin and glucose response in vivo and in vitro in patients with coronary heart disease." *Metabolism* 45:669–72.

Frost, G., G. Trew, R. Margara, A. R. Leeds, A. Dornhorst. 1998. "Improvement in adipocyte insulin response to low glycemic index diet in women at risk of cardiovascular disease." *Metabolism* 47:1245–51.

Giacco, R., M. Parillo, A. A. Rivellese, G. Lasorella, A. Giacco, L. D'episcopo, and G. Riccardi. 2000. "Long-term dietary treatment with increased amounts of fibre-rich low-glycemic index natural foods improves blood glucose control and reduces the number of hypoglycemic events in type 1 diabetic patients." *Diabetes Care* 23:1461–66.

Gilbertson, H. R., J. C. Brand-Miller, A. W. Thorburn, S. Evans, P. Chondros, and G. A. Werther. 2001. "The effect of flexible low glycemic index dietary advice versus measured carbohydrate exchange diets on glycemic control in children with type 1 diabetes." *Diabetes Care* 24:1137–43.

Hu, F., and B. W. C. Willett. 2002. "Optimal diets for prevention of coronary heart disease." *Journal of the American Medical Association* 288(20) (Nov. 27): 2569–78.

Jenkins, D. J. A., L. S. A. Augustin, C. W. C. Kendall, et al. 2002. "Glycemic index: overview of implications in health and disease." *American Journal of Clinical Nutrition* 76:266S–273S.

Jenkins, D. J. A., T. M. S. Wolever, R.H., Taylor, et al. 1981. "Glycemic index of foods: A physiological basis for carbohydrate exchange." *American Journal of Clinical Nutrition* 34:362–66.

Jenkins, D. J., M. Axelsen, C. W. Kendall, L. S. Augustin, V. Vuksan, and U. Smith. 2000. "Dietary fibre, lente carbohydrates and the insulin-resistant diseases." *British Journal of Nutrition* 83(1) (March): S157–63.

Fernandes, G., A. Velangi, and T. M. S. Wolever. 2005. "Glycemic index of potatoes commonly consumed in North America." *Journal of the American Dietetic Association* 105(4):557–62.

Kelly, S., G. Frost, V. Whittaker, and C. Summerbell. 2004. "Low glycemic index diets for coronary heart disease." *Cochrane Database of Systemic Reviews* (4) (Oct. 18): CD004467.

Leeds, A. R. 2002. "Glycemic index and heart disease." *American Journal of Clinical Nutrition* 76 (1)(July): 286S–9S.

Leeman, M., E. Ostman, and I. Bjorck. 2005. Vinegar dressing and cold storage of potatoes lowers postprandial glycaemic and insulinaemic responses in healthy subjects. *European Journal of Clinical Nutrition*. 59(11):1266–71.

Liu, S., J. E. Manson, J. E. Buring, M. J. Stampfer, W. C. Willett, and P. M. Ridker. 2002. "Relation between a diet with a high glycemic load and plasma concentrations of high-sensitivity C-reactive protein in middle-aged women." *American Journal of Clinical Nutrition* 75:492–98.

Liu, S., J. E. Manson, M. J. Stampfer, M. D. Holmes, F. B. Hu, S. E. Hankinson, and W. C. Willett. 2001. "Dietary glycemic load assessed by food-frequency questionnaire in relation to plasma high-density-lipoprotein cholesterol and fasting plasma triacylglycerols in postmenopausal women." *American Journal of Clinical Nutrition* 73:560–66.

Liu, S., M., J. Stampfer, J. E. Manson, F. B. Ju, M. Franz, C. H. Hennekens, and W. C. Willet. 1998. "A prospective study of dietary glycemic load and risk of myocardial infarction in women." *Federation of American Societies for Experimental Biology Journal* 124: A260 (abstract#1517).

Liu, S., W. C. Willett, M. J. Stampfer, F. B. Hu, M. Franz, L. Sampson, C. H. Hennekens, and J. E. Manson. 2000. "A prospective study of dietary glycemic load, carbohydrate intake and risk of coronary heart disease in US women." *American Journal of Clinical Nutrition* 71:1455–61.

Liu, S., W. C. Willett. 2002. "Dietary glycemic load and atherothrombotic risk." *Current Atherosclerosis Reports* 4(6) (Nov.): 454–61.

Ludwig, D. S. 2000. "Dietary glycemic index and obesity." *Journal of Nutrition* 130:280S–283S.

———2002. "The glycemic index. Physiological mechanisms relating to obesity, diabetes, and cardiovascular disease." *Journal of the American Medical Association* 287:2414–23.

Ludwig, D. S. and R. H. Eckel. 2002. "The glycemic index at 20y." *American Journal of Clinical Nutrition* 76:264S–265S.

Ludwig, D. S., J. A. Majzoub, A. Al-Zahrani, G. E. Dallal, I. Blanco, and S. B. Roberts. 1999. "High glycemic index foods, overeating, and obesity." *Pediatrics* 103(3).

McKeown, N. M., J. B. Meigs, S. Liu, E. Saltzman, P. W. Wilson, and P. F. Jacques. 2004. "Carbohydrate nutrition, insulin resistance, and the prevalence of the metabolic syndrome in the Framingham Offspring Cohort." *Diabetes Care* 27(2) (Feb.): 538–46.

McMillan-Price, J., P. Petocz, F. Atkinson, K. O'Neill, S. Samman, K. Steinbeck, I. Caterson, and J. Brand-Miller. 2006. "Comparison of four diets of varying glycemic load on weight loss and cardiovascular risk reduction in overweight and obese young adults." *Archives of Internal Medicine* 166: 1466–1475.

McMillan-Price, J.,and J. Brand-Miller. 2004. "Dietary approaches to overweight and obesity." *American Journal of Clinical Dermatology* 22(4) (Jul.-Aug.): 310–14.

Moses, R. G., M. Luebcke, W. S. Davis, K. J. Coleman, L. C. Tapsell, P. Petocz, and J. C. Brand-Miller. 2006. "Effect of a low-glycemic-index diet during pregnancy on obstetric outcomes." *American Journal of Clinical Nutrition* 84: 807–812.National Health and Medical Research Council. 1999. "Dietary Guidelines for Older Australians." *Ausinfo*, Canberra.

Patel, V. C., R. D. Aldridge, A. Leeds, A. Dornhorst, and G. S. Frost. 2004. "Retrospective analysis of the impact of a low glycemic index diet on hospital stay following coronary artery bypass grafting: A hypothesis." *Journal of Human Nutrition and Dietetics* 17(3) (June): 241–47.

Pi-Sunyer, F. X. 2002. "Glycemic index and disease." *American Journal of Clinical Nutrition* 76:290S–298S.

Position Statement by the Canadian Diabetes Association. 1999. "Guidelines for the nutritional management of diabetes mellitus in the new millennium." *Canadian Journal of Diabetes Care* 23(3):56–69.

Salmeron, J., E. B. Ascherio, G. A. Rimm, D. Colditz, D. Spiegelman, D. J. Jenkins, M. J. Stampfer, A. A. Wing, and W. C. Willet. 1997. "Dietary fiber, glycemic load and risk of NIDDM in men." *Diabetes Care* 20:545–50.

Salmeron, J., J. E. Manson, M. J. Stampfer, G. A. Colditz, A. L. Wing, and W. C. Willet. 1997. "Dietary fiber, glycemic load and risk of non-insulin-dependent diabetes mellitus in women." *Journal of the American Medical Association* 277:472–77.

Skurk, T., and H. Hauner. 2004. "Obesity and impaired fibrinolysis: Role of adipose production of plasminogen activator inhibitor-1." *International Journal of Obesity and Related Metabolic Disorders* 28(11) (Nov.): 1357–64.

Spieth, L. E., J. D. Harnish, C. M. Lenders, L. B. Raezer, M. A. Pereira, J. Hangen, and D. S. Ludwig. 2000. "A low-glycemic index diet in the treatment of pediatric obesity." *Archives of Pediatric and Adolescent Medicine* 154:947–51.

Trayhurn, P., and I. S. Wood. 2004. "Adipokines: Inflammation and the pleiotropic role of white adipose tissue." *British Journal of Nutrition* 92(3) (Sept.): 347–55.

Wilkin, T. J., and L. D. Voss. 2004. "Metabolic syndrome: Maladaptation to a modern world." *Journal of the Royal Society of Medicine* 97(11) (Nov.): 511–20.

Willett, W., J. Manson, and S. Liu. 2002. "Glycemic index, glycemic load, and risk of type 2 diabetes." *American Journal of Clinical Nutrition* 76: 274S–280S.

Wolever, T. M. S., M. Yang, X. Y. Zeng, F. Atkinson, and J. C. Brand-Miller. 2006. "Food glycemic index, as given in Glycemic Index tables, is a significant determinant of glycemic responses elicited by composite breakfast meals. *American Journal of Clinical Nutrition.* 83(6):1306–12.

Low-GI Foods and Weight:
A Summary of the Scientific Evidence

Country	Subjects	Study design	Findings	Reference details
Australia	Overweight young adults	89 subjects followed 1 of 4 diets for 12 weeks (1) produced around standard low-fat; (2) low-GI; (3) higher protein; (4) low-GI and protein	Compared with the standard low-fat diet, all 3 modified diets improved findings, 2004. 50% more fat loss. Risk factors for heart disease improved more on the low-GI diet.	McMillan-Price et al., *Archives of Internal Medicine*, 2006
USA	Overweight young adults	39 subjects consumed a low-GI or low-fat diet to achieve a 10% weight loss in both groups	Resting metabolic rate declined less in the low-GI group (-6%) than the low-fat group (-11%). Risk factors for heart disease improved more on the low-GI diet.	Pereira et al., in press
USA	Overweight adolescents	16 subjects followed a low-fat diet or a low-glycemic load diet for 12 months	Those who followed the low-GL diet lost more body fat and kept it off. The low-fat group gained body fat during the second 6 months.	Ebbeling et al., *Archives of Pediatric and Adolescent Medicine*, 2003
UK	Overweight men	17 men consumed 1 of 4 diets for 24 days	Despite efforts to maintain identical energy intake, men on the low-GI diet lost weight compared with those on the high-GI, high-fat, and high-sugar diets.	Byrnes et al., *British Journal of Nutrition*, 2003.
France	Overweight men	11 subjects followed high or low-GI diets for 5 weeks each without aiming to lose weight	During the low GI perod, the men lost 500 g of body fat from around the waist.	Bouche et al, *Diabetes Care*, 2003
USA	Overweight children	109 children consumed either a low-GI or a conventional low fat diet for 4 months	17% of the children in the low-GI group achieved a 3-unit decrease in body mass index, compared with only 2% in the low-fat group.	Spieth et al, *Archives of Pediatric and Adolescent Medicine*, 2000

Country	Subjects	Study design	Findings	Reference details
Germany	Adults with type 1 diabetes	Cross-sectional study with 1500 adults in 31 clinics across Europe	The GI of the diet correlated positively with waist circumference in men.	Buyken et al, *International Journal of Obesity*, 2001
USA	Pregnant women	12 women ate a high- or low-GI diet during pregnancy	Those on the low-GI diet gained 12 kg compared with 20 kg in women on the high GI diet.	Clapp J, *Archives of Gynaecology and Obstetrics*, 1997
South Africa	Overweight women	30 women consumed a high- or low-GI diet for two 12-week periods	Those on the low-GI diet lost 2 kg more in the first 12 weeks and then 3 kg more in the second 12.	Slabber et al, *American Journal of Clinical Nutrition*, 1994

Acknowledgments

*M*any people have contributed to the third North American edition of *The New Glucose Revolution* and its predecessors in the New Glucose Revolution series, and we are most grateful to them all.

Firstly, we would like to acknowledge and thank our colleagues who contributed to particular chapters in this edition: Joanna McMillan-Price (chapter 6), Anthony Leeds (chapter 9), Professor Nadir R. Farid (chapter 10), Kate Marsh (chapters 10 and 15), Heather Gilbertson (chapter 11), Helen O' Connor (chapter 12), Philippa Sandall (chapters 15 and 16) and Lisa Lintner who created a number of recipes especially for us (pages 263–266, 280, and 292).

We are deeply indebted to our tireless publisher, Matthew Lore, for his passion, commitment, and attention to every detail. This edition would not have happened without his support. Of course we know he has the backing of a great team at Marlowe & Company and we'd especially like to thank Courtney Napoles, Vince Kunkemueller, Kathryn McHugh, Linda Kosarin, and Jonathan Sainsbury.

Our thanks also to Kathleen Hanuschak, for her work on the recipes in part 4 and the tables in part 5; Camille Noe Pagán, for her many editorial contributions; Ann Kirschner, for her meticulous copyediting; Pauline Neuwirth, for her book design and typesetting; and Michael Fusco, for his series cover design.

We are most grateful to Catherine Saxelby, who got us off to a good start when we first decided we wanted to write a book about the glycemic index; Philippa Sandall, our literary agent, who has contributed to the success of all the books in the series; and to all those who have supported the GI approach and recommended our books, particularly Diabetes Australia and the Juvenile Diabetes Research Foundation.

Many dietitians, doctors, colleagues, and readers have given us feedback and played a large role in the success of the series, some of whom deserve special mention: Shirley Crossman, Martina Chippendall, Helen O'Connor, Heather Gilbertson, Alan Barclay, Rudi Bartl, Kate Marsh, Toni Irwin, David Jenkins, David Ludwig, Simin Liu, Ted Arnold, Warren Kidson, Bob Moses, Ian Caterson, Stewart Truswell, Gareth Denyer, Fiona Atkinson, Scott Dickinson, Joanna McMillan-Price, Johanna Burani, and David Mendosa.

Lastly, we thank our wonderful, long-suffering partners, John Miller, Judy Wolever, Jonathan Powell, and Ruth Colagiuri, respectively, for all those nights and weekends when we were otherwise occupied.

Index

Recipe Index

Meet the Medical Doctors, Scientists, and Clinicians Behind the All-New Third Edition of *The New Glucose Revolution*

JENNIE BRAND-MILLER, PhD, is one of the world's foremost authorities on carbohydrates and the glycemic index and has championed the GI approach to nutrition for more than twenty-five years. Professor of Nutrition at the University of Sydney and the immediate past president of the Nutrition Society of Australia, Brand-Miller manages a GI food-labeling program in Australia (www.gisymbol.com.au) with Diabetes Australia and the Juvenile Diabetes Research Foundation to ensure that claims about the GI are scientifically correct and are applied only to nutritious foods. Winner of Australia's prestigious ATSE Clunies Ross Award in 2003 for her commitment to advancing science and technology, Brand-Miller is an in-demand speaker, and her laboratory at the University of Sydney is recognized worldwide for cutting-edge research on carbohydrates and health.

THOMAS M. S. WOLEVER, MD, is professor in the Department of Nutritional Sciences, University of Toronto, and a member of the Division of Endocrinology and Metabolism, St. Michael's Hospital, Toronto. He is a graduate of Oxford University (BA, MA, MB, B.Ch, M.Sc, and DM) in the United Kingdom. He received his PhD at the University of Toronto.

Since 1980, his research has focused on the glycemic index of foods and the prevention of type 2 diabetes. The coauthor of other books in the New Glucose Revolution series, he lives in Toronto, Canada.

KAYE FOSTER-POWELL, M NUTR & DIET, an accredited dietitian-nutritionist with extensive experience in diabetes management, counsels hundreds of people a year on how to improve their health and well-being and reduce their risk of diabetic complications through a low-GI diet. Foster-Powell is the coauthor with Jennie Brand-Miller of all books in the New Glucose Revolution series, as well as of the authoritative tables of GI and glycemic load values published in the *American Journal of Clinical Nutrition*.

STEPHEN COLAGIURI, MD, is the director of the Diabetes Center and head of the Department of Endocrinology, Metabolism, and Diabetes at the Prince of Wales Hospital in Randwick, New South Wales, Australia. He graduated from the University of Sydney and is a Fellow of the Royal Australasian College of Physicians. He has a joint academic appointment at the University of New South Wales. He has more than one hundred scientific papers to his name, many concerned with the importance of carbohydrates in the diet of people with diabetes, and is coauthor of many books in the New Glucose Revolution series.